Breaking Eggs

*Finding New Meaning
with Chronic Illness*

LUCIA AMSDEN

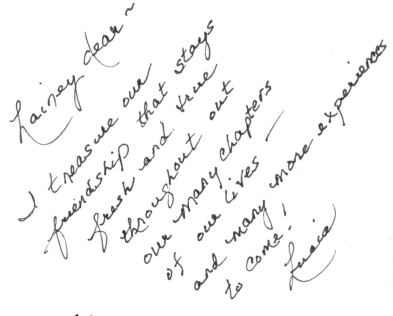

Lainey dear~
I treasure our stays
friendship that stays
fresh and true
throughout our
our many chapters
of our lives
and many more experiences
to come!
Lucia

outskirtspress
DENVER, COLORADO

Outskirts Press, Inc.
http://www.outskirtspress.com

ISBN: 978-1-4327-9610-5

Library of Congress Control Number: 2012946857

Outskirts Press and the "OP" logo are trademarks belonging to Outskirts Press, Inc.

PRINTED IN THE UNITED STATES OF AMERICA

"It's a chance to give new meaning to every move we make"

NEIL YOUNG, FROM THE SONG, "LIGHT A CANDLE"

Contents

Acknowledgements

*T*hank you to my amazing husband, Tim Amsden, and my spiritual teacher and friend, Deborah Singleton. The healing vision of health and well-being they have always carried for me has become my own.

To friends and family for your encouragement and helpful nudges. I know some of you wondered at times if I would ever complete this book. Your encouraging words kept me going.

To the people who so generously provided their own stories to be included in *Breaking Eggs*. Your shared experiences and lessons added great depth and wisdom to understanding what it means to deal with chronic illness.

To those who read the manuscript and gave me editorial comments and feedback that clarified and energized ideas. You helped it all come together.

And finally, to you who are holding this book in your hands at this moment. You were in the room, invisible but very present, as I wrote my story. This book is dedicated to you and your search for new meaning in your life.

My new meaning is that we are all truly One.

Lucia Amsden

Foreword

While I sit writing this, I smile and think back to the day I first met Lucia. I was conducting a seminar on healing in Kansas City, and afterwards I did some healing work with individual clients. Lucia was not able to attend the seminar, but booked a private appointment. I remember her well, coming to meet with me. Fragile and thin, holding her energy so close for fear of losing what she had of it, but the most profound observation was the beautiful light from her eyes. That was an indication to me that even though her prognosis was not good, she was determined, her spirit was bright and strong, and she was looking for a way to heal.

Breaking Eggs: Finding New Meaning with Chronic Illness is a genuine story of healing and hope. As on any journey, whether it is a chronic illness or a desire to change one's life, it begins with a decision and a step forward. The path to change is rarely straight. It is in keeping the destination in the mind's eye that the roadblocks become opportunities to learn, and the crossroads are places to pause and decide what is truly desired. Lucia shares the twists and turns of her journey with engaging stories of her personal journey, as well as stories of others who are also healing.

Lucia invites you to explore your innate power of transformation and regeneration for physical, as well as emotional and spiritual health. Throughout these pages you will find ways to awaken your heart and mind to new depths of truth. You can learn how to quiet your mind and connect to your inner guidance, and move toward an attitude of compassion and gratitude and a knowing that the body is a gift to be treasured.

This book offers a delightful and practical guide for working with the challenges of illness while supporting your daily life. You will find an inspiring message of hope, courage, and the demonstration of self-healing through simple yet powerful tools. There is a message of absolute acceptance of oneself, to forgive the past and tap into innate healing abilities that are a basic part of human nature.

To give one's self to healing is a beautiful and thrilling commitment. It takes great courage to retreat to the innocence of the soul, as well as touch both intelligence and worldly wisdom, and use them all to heal. As a friend and co-traveler on this life path, I am honored and privileged to be a part of Lucia's process toward health. It has been said that a miracle is a change in perception. We have a miracle here!

Deborah Singleton
President, Arasini Foundation
Director, A Healing Place
Dallas, Texas

Introduction

> "All journeys have secret destinations of
> which the traveler is unaware."
>
> MARTIN BUBER

Some distance behind our house is a labyrinth, laid out with rough fieldstones, nestled within a circle of tall Ponderosa Pines. I have regularly walked its winding path for the last ten years. It has particular meaning for me because it symbolizes a journey I began thirty years ago, when as a young woman I was diagnosed with rheumatoid arthritis.

Labyrinths are intentionally confounding. They turn and circle in and out. Just as you seem to be moving toward the center, out you go again. They are, however, different from mazes. Mazes are full of false turns and dead ends. Labyrinths contain only one path, which will carry you unerringly to the center.

At the heart of my labyrinth is a bench made of slabs of sandstone. At its base rests a large heart-shaped rock, a tangible symbol of the heart of this sacred place. Beneath the seat is a bowl filled with pottery shards and glass hearts, gifts for friends who come and walk the path when we're not here. Scattered on the bench are gifts some of them have left—crystals, a tiny glass Earth, a shell, small crosses.

Labyrinths have been around for thousands of years. They endure because circling along their paths without any mental map of how they connect to the center, encourages the mind to release control and the heart to trust. When these things happen we feel more free of fears and resentments. We open to the gentle voice of our spirit. This is also what I have tried to do as I walk the greater labyrinth of my life with illness.

For many of us, the beginning of our journey with chronic illness seems like a maze, filled with confusing paths and stumbles toward dead ends. With time and intent, however, the things we learn and experience can transform our journey so that it becomes more like a labyrinth. We can learn to profoundly trust our path. We can develop a stronger sense of our hearts. Despite apparent diversions and setbacks, we can move in healing spirals into our spirits.

The book you're holding in your hands is not about curing your body of illness, though that may happen. It is about your healing path, your own journey toward integrating all your physical, emotional, mental, and especially your spiritual aspects. It is about living more peacefully.

Even as we grieve for what we've lost, we can be moving into our spiritual nature. When our primary focus shifts from our disease to our healing journey, we create a sanctuary within ourselves; a place where we love more, nourish our spirits, and dwell more in our hearts where true healing can occur.

In the following pages I offer my healing journey along with stories of others living with their challenges, and lay out some of the principles and tools that have helped me move toward a life more focused on my authentic self. I hope they will help you along your own path.

———— ⊗⊗⊗ ————

I invite you to trace with your finger the labyrinth path at the end of this Introduction. Clear your mind, slow and deepen your breath, and allow your body to relax. Slide your finger into the labyrinth entrance and allow it to slowly follow the path, as if you were meandering through a large labyrinth in a grassy field. As your finger wends its way in and out and in again, allow yourself to begin releasing something you no longer wish to carry in your life. Pause at the center of the labyrinth and breathe into the light empty space you are creating. Move slowly back toward the entrance, bringing lightness and clarity with you.

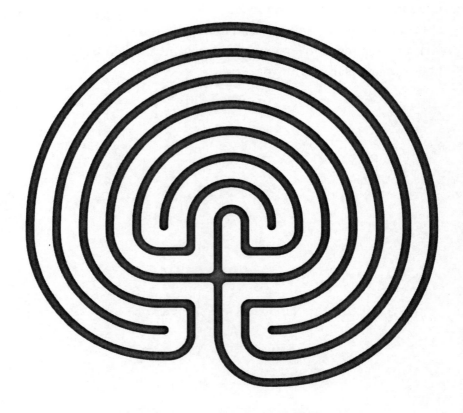

Classic Seven Circuit Labyrinth

Thanks to Labyrinthos, www.labyrinthos.com,
for permission to use the illustration.

CHAPTER 1

The Journey Begins

"Meaning helps us see in the dark."

RACHEL NAOMI RAMEN

I still remember it as if it were yesterday— sitting on a cold metal table, waiting for the doctor to come in with my test results. I was in a standard antiseptic room with a generic calendar on the wall, samples of unknown medicines, and a chrome stool. I felt tense all over, as if I were bracing myself against some unknown threat. As I waited, I tried to calm myself.

I reviewed what had brought me to this moment. A few months earlier I'd been struggling with a swollen knee that I ascribed to a fall during a ski trip. But as my pain spread to my shoulders and feet, I knew something was definitely wrong that had nothing to do with skiing. My body felt completely out of control, as each day brought more pain and discomfort. I finally decided that it was time to find out what was wrong.

The doctor came in and sat on the stool with the test results on his lap. I heard him tell me that I had rheumatoid arthritis, a disease of the joints. He went on to say that there was no known cure; it was a chronic condition that I would have for the rest of my life. I even recall what I was thinking about as the doctor's voice droned on. I flashed to a picture of my stepmother crippled with rheumatoid arthritis, finally dying of complications from the disease. I saw her using her walker and sitting in a chair lift to get to the second floor of our house. Most of all, I remember her face full of pain and anger at what her body was doing to her.

As I tuned back in to what the doctor was saying, I heard him talk about limiting my activities, resting twice a day, and curtailing my busy life. It was a foreign concept to someone who had two young sons and who saw cramming as much as possible into each day as a competitive game. I asked the doctor about my last year of graduate school in social work, which was to begin in a few weeks. He discouraged finishing my degree, saying it would be too demanding, and suggested I also stop yoga because it would hurt my joints.

As I left the doctor's office on that September afternoon, I realized that my thirty-seven-year-old world as I knew it had ended. I felt completely alone, standing on a faultline that rumbled and split wide beneath my feet.

Not too long ago, I talked to one of my sons about that period. Ten years old at the time, he said he remembered my coming home, crying, and telling him I had a disease called rheumatoid arthritis. He also remembered his dad later saying that he and his brother would have to help more around the house. For me, that early time is a complete blur of pain.

Even though the doctor had advised against finishing graduate school, after some thought I decided to go ahead. Somehow I intuitively knew that continuing my schooling would be good for me mentally and emotionally, even if it would be a physical struggle. It was the first sign that I would learn to follow my intuition, even when no one agreed with me. In hindsight, it was the best thing I could have done for myself.

That year I attended a presentation by Elizabeth Kubler-Ross, a famous researcher and author on death and dying, who was a guest speaker at the medical center where I was taking my course work. Her quiet and assuring voice reached out to me through the fog and confusion of that time. She said that people suffering a major loss of any kind usually go in and out of predictable emotional stages of shock, denial, bargaining, anger, depression, acceptance, and hope.

Her words touched me deeply as I struggled with my own losses from the onset of arthritis. It was a relief to realize that I was in the middle of a natural process, and that I could expect things to get better. I understood that I wasn't yet at the stages of acceptance or hope, but that I was in the midst of working through the stages that went before. She helped me make sense of all my confusing feelings.

Later as I mulled over her presentation, I realized that I was especially locked in the emotional stage of anger. My anger would come out in small ways, such as getting mad at a slow driver in front of me or wanting to throw a tightly closed jar across the kitchen. What surprised me was that my anger also fueled certain healthy actions.

Shortly after her presentation, I attended a meeting at a local hospital for patients suffering from chronic illness. A well-known rheumatologist was the main speaker for the evening. The hospital conference room was packed full of people with a range of chronic conditions. What I remember most about the presentation was a series of slides graphically portraying people in advanced stages of several diseases, from multiple sclerosis to rheumatoid arthritis. There were pictures of people with severely deformed spines, twisted hands, and other physical deformities. The speaker approached the audience as if he were lecturing to a group of doctors who were clinically studying advanced stages of various diseases.

After the program, I remember stepping into an elevator and seeing it full of people looking as shell-shocked as I. It was clear that rather than being helpful, those pictures added to our fears.

After some thought, I wrote the physician a letter sharing my concerns about his presentation, and eventually received a fairly defensive reply. The important thing to me, though, was not how he received my note, but the fact that I took the action of writing to an authority figure at all. It was an action I would not have taken in the past. Throughout my life I had suppressed anger. But I was beginning to find my voice and speak up.

Although it was good to have a framework for what I was going through, mentally understanding the stages of loss was wholly different than deeply experiencing the emotions. I was profoundly depressed, and my thoughts about myself became increasingly negative. I felt as if my life had been stripped away.

I was becoming very limited in what I could physically do. I dreaded mornings the most, when the pain was particularly severe and my young family needed me. Lifting, bending, and even walking had become a labor. The sports that had given me such pleasure and that had helped me manage my stress were gone from my life. I often brooded that I could no longer be the mother and wife that I thought I should be. The world around me was going about its business as usual, but I had become so different.

My husband and I were growing more and more distant from each other. We'd put all our focus and energy on trying to be good parents, and had not built a strong foundation between us that would help us weather a life-altering disease. Distance and misunderstandings multiplied, and after twenty years we finally realized that our marriage was over.

My relationship with my two sons was the most important thing in my life, but what use was I to them? My new social work career seemed like too much effort. Why stay around? I was going downhill fast. Why not let the pain and sadness take over, just as I had seen it do to my stepmother? It was my darkest hour.

During this lonely time, despite my hopelessness and depression, I felt a healthy spark slowly start to grow. I didn't know then what it was, but I know now my soul was giving me comfort and courage to carry on. I was slowly realizing that at my core I am a spiritual being untouched by illness. My spirit was gradually emerging to guide me through this hard, gritty time that was turning my life upside down.

That diagnosis handed to me by my doctor, laden with all his knowledge and power, seemed final and certain. He told me that I would always have this disease, that I had to be careful about what I did, and that I should avoid pushing myself. He was dispensing words and ideas that limited the rest of my life. I can't remember another time when I was so subject to someone else's influence.

Our diagnosis comes at a time when many of us are most vulnerable to what the medical system predicts and prescribes. The name of a condition is instantly placed like a weight upon our shoulders, and we are told how our life will change.

Our physician will probably tell us what the progress of the disease will be, based on his or her training and experience. He or she may stress the challenges and difficulties ahead, wanting us to truly understand and prepare for what they see as inevitable. For many of us it is a deeply defining moment, an instant when our lives become something else, something scary and reduced from what we were a second before.

I don't want to give the impression that all doctors deliver diagnoses this way—some, hopefully many, tell patients the nature of their disorders more softly, with an understanding of the impact of their words. They realize that their knowledge is limited, so they talk in terms of possibilities. They leave room for the patient to grow and heal in ways that may not fit into the Western medical model.

If only we could all receive our diagnosis with an understanding that the doctor is only one expert, operating only in the realm of Western medicine. We, not they, are in charge of our lives, and we have access to many resources outside the tradition of the medical community, the most important being ourselves. Rather than receiving the diagnosis like baby birds, we'd be much better (I would have been so much better) if we'd take these medical predictions and recommendations with a grain of salt, allowing us space to be the authors of our own stories.

It is helpful to me to understand where doctors are often coming from. They want the patient to take their diagnosis seriously, so that the patient takes the steps they believe to be best from a medical standpoint. This may lead them to speak especially authoritatively and assertively.

Also, they are experts—they are highly trained and usually have long experience with diagnosing the disease they ascribe to us. Sometimes this can lead them to false certainty about where our disorders will lead us.

I once went to a rheumatologist who examined my hands and remarked that I suffered a great deal of pain. I told him that although I had suffered significant pain in the past, I had been fairly pain free for a long time. "No," he said, "I can see from your hands that you have a great deal of pain." Doctors may sometimes assert their expertise in denial of your right to your own physical situation and even, sometimes, of your own history.

If I could have gone into my diagnosis with an understanding of the limitations of the medical field, with the knowledge that I'm much more than my diagnosis, I would not have been quite so devastated by the doctor's words. If I could have tempered what he was saying with awareness of the spiritual and other resources around and within me, and a conviction that my story is mine alone to write, I could have saved myself a great deal of suffering. But that's not the way these events usually happen. It's only later, after the diagnosis, that we gradually discover who and what we really are.

To make matters worse, I added to my own distress by imagining the direst consequences. Even though I knew that rheumatoid arthritis was rarely a fatal disease, my mind rushed to the scariest scenario. I was immediately immersed in images of my stepmother, as I watched her slow anguished death. I saw myself going through the same awful process.

Irrespective of how it is delivered, a diagnosis places us in a category for which we assume we will all have similar outcomes. It's taken me a long time to become aware of how I allowed memories of what happened to my stepmother to worsen my own situation.

Now I do much better. When I remember my stepmother's difficult death or see someone wrestle with the challenges of severe arthritis, I gently remind myself that their experiences and mine are not identical. Each of us follows a unique and different path, and it's important to realize that we are much more than our disease.

Depending on the nature and severity of our illness, it's easy to lose ourselves in it. We can even define ourselves by it. If we are not careful, being ill can dominate our thinking, what we talk about, and how we behave. In fact, the very nature of the English language supports labeling ourselves by our illnesses. We say "I am a diabetic," for instance, rather than referring to ourselves as people with diabetes.

This is another area where the medical community could be more helpful. Once, as an orthopedic surgeon was looking at an x-ray of my hand, he said, "Arthritics have hands that..." I told him I would prefer that he not refer to me as an arthritic, but rather describe me as a person who has arthritis. I don't think he understood what I was trying to say, because within a short time he referred to me once again as an arthritic.

Sometimes I want to shout, "Remember, there's a person behind this illness." Particularly in those early days, I needed to continually remind myself of that fact.

There are people who come into our lives to teach us important lessons. As a counselor, when a new client walked through my door I would often say to myself, "I wonder what new lessons he or she has for me?" I had a client whom I'll call Alice, who clearly showed me what happens when a physical illness overtakes everything else.

At her first visit, Alice immediately began describing the nightmare of her past five years with fibromyalgia and all her problems with doctors, pain specialists, and psychologists. With relish she gave example after example of how she never got straight answers from medical people. One of her doctors even "fired" her, by telling her she should find someone else.

Alice complained that in other areas of her life, things weren't going much better. Her children and grandchildren were busy with their lives and uninterested in her health problems. When her husband was at home, he spent most of his time on the computer and paid little attention to her. She had lost interest in her garden because it was too difficult to keep up with, and she had stopped pursuing most of her other interests such as writing poetry and seeing friends, because she didn't have the energy.

Alice admitted she felt helpless and depressed much of the time. She was taking an anti-depressant and had recently gone through a six-week program at a pain clinic. As I sat in my office listening to her story, I wondered if our counseling would be another revolving door through which she would soon move.

From her perspective, the more she searched for help, the more things stayed the same or got worse. It became clear that Alice held a firm belief that no one understood her or cared about her pain. I could see that it was taking enormous energy for her to prove to me and to anyone else who would listen, what a victim she was of this terrible disease.

Over the next few months, I met a few members of her family. It was clear that they didn't know how to treat this once gregarious and outgoing person who had turned into an angry and distant stranger.

As our sessions continued, Alice slowly started to make an effort to reconnect with her adult children. She went on several shopping outings with her daughter and enjoyed a family gathering. She grudgingly admitted that she was monitoring herself and trying not to constantly complain to her husband and others about her pain. Her life seemed to be getting brighter as she became more a participant again in the world around her.

Alice once told me that when she was a youngster, her parents had been in a serious automobile accident. Her mother had suffered from severe physical problems for several years afterward. As we delved into those early years, Alice realized that at some point she had begun to feel that her world wasn't safe. If this terrible thing could happen to her parents, what unforeseen catastrophes might happen to her?

Alice's childhood feelings of helplessness were battling with an emerging belief that she didn't have to be a victim of her fibromyalgia. But her sense of helplessness was too ingrained—the way her illness struck her out of the blue was not that different from the way her parents' accident had turned her young world upside down.

She gradually started canceling her appointments with me. In the last few sessions, she talked about how my counseling wasn't giving her any benefit. She admitted that she felt better when she re-engaged with her family, but would not admit that her positive efforts improved her overall well-being. She finally quit coming to our counseling sessions completely.

All the work Alice did, though, wasn't futile. For a time, she experienced what it was like to re-inhabit her life. For a short period, her illness wasn't defining her. I like to think that, although the positive changes she experienced had been put aside, they will be available to her whenever she decides to try again.

We're our own storytellers. Each of us has a story related to our illness that is both unique and woven of common threads. Our story governs how we see our current situation, and it is a framework that supports or limits our future possibilities. It's important that we become aware of the power of our stories to shape our thoughts, words, and pictures. As we do, we take important first steps toward developing healthy attitudes, so we do not live mired in anger and depression.

When chronic illness enters our lives, we all experience times of anger, sadness, depression, and grief. This is normal and even healthy—anger, for instance, can be a very useful tool for motivating us to change. We don't have to remain there, though. We have a choice to move toward greater acceptance and hope.

When we actively commit to a strong undercurrent of hope, we step out of the prison of the illness box. Our primary focus shifts from the disease in our bodies to living a richer, more meaningful life. We move toward living our lives as people, not diseases.

CHAPTER 2

Looking Fear in the Eye

"The only way around something is through it."

I can still remember the embarrassment I felt as a young teen-ager, watching cloth pads that I'd used to fill out the top of my swimsuit come floating to the surface. The pads slipped out when I'd dived into the pool, and now bobbed like small saucers on top of the water. Imagine the laughter and teasing that went on among the kids in the pool. Several of the boys had great fun acting as if they were playing volleyball, throwing the pads back and forth. Fortunately they'd surfaced a good distance from where I was swimming, so I didn't have to admit they were mine.

As a young person I always felt that my body didn't measure up to those of my friends. When someone teased me about being underdeveloped, it really hurt. In retrospect there actually wasn't very much teasing, but I took to heart the small amount that came my way. At the time I had no idea that the pattern I was developing of being critical of my body would be with me for a long time.

The swimming pool incident was a small thing, something most of us would forget quickly, but it popped into my mind many years later when I was pondering the critical attitudes I carried about my body. I had one of those "aha" experiences, realizing that my tendency to reprimand myself for having a body that didn't measure up was going strong even when I was a teen-ager, when I often compared my body's shape to those of others. Over the years I had further expanded my repertoire of judgments, not only criticizing my shape but also hammering away at my lack of energy and my inability to do all I wanted or thought I should do. Now with arthritis, those negative thoughts were stronger than ever.

I gradually became aware that my negative attitudes about my body affected me in many ways. In addition to contributing to my general feelings of not measuring up to those around me, they depleted my vitality. They drained my energy and sapped my will to get better.

As I worked deeper into my unhealthy attitudes about my body, my mind went back to my adolescence when I pushed myself hard in basketball, tennis, and other activities without any consideration of whether it was good for me. When I was young, I'd work myself to such a pitch that I would sometimes get physically ill. Then I'd head to bed to recover, catch up on sleep, and hide under the pillow to momentarily keep the world at bay.

I discovered early on, as most kids do, that when I was sick I received special care. Being sick was also a way to get out of things. Pushing myself until I was ill gave me a good excuse for delaying turning in a project, or not having to face some other problem at school.

I thought about episodes I experienced with stomach problems many years ago, and a six-year bout of hives. Throughout my life, my body has been sending me clear messages that it needed love and care, but I didn't know how to listen. I treated my body as a machine that I expected to run forever and when it failed temporarily, I used it to get out of things I didn't want to do.

In addition to being critical, fear about my body also began early. The fear took strong root when I was about eleven, as I watched my mother die slowly of colon cancer over a two-year period. I didn't understand what was happening—people around me didn't talk openly about what my mother was going through. Cancer was a hush-hush subject. It's hard to believe now, but I didn't even know she had cancer until I overheard it mentioned after her funeral. All I knew was that she was seriously ill and went to a hospital often, and that I was slowly losing her.

In our family we didn't know how to share our fears and worries with each other. I believe my dad felt that it was important to appear strong and steady for my sister and me, and it would have shown weakness for him to talk about feelings and the emotional pain that was heavy in the air.

I don't want to give the impression that there weren't loving and caring people in our family and in our community. I remember one particular evening service when our church congregation prayed for my mother's recovery. But I felt alone, without a safe place where I could let my tears fall.

I can't imagine how hard it must have been for my mother. She had a good friend who visited her often, but for the most part I think she felt isolated from others, ashamed and terrified about what was happening to her body.

I vividly remember one day when I came home from school, and as I always did, went into her room. I can still see her in bed beside the double windows in the late afternoon light. As I sat next to her on her bed, she looked over at me and remarked wistfully how much she wished she were healthy so she could be the mother she wanted to be.

In that moment I was overcome with an intense yearning to make her well. At the same time I helplessly knew there was nothing I could do. Whatever was happening to her body was a force to be feared. I believe I took that contagious fear into myself.

About a year after my mother's death, a very close family friend who lived next door died of cancer. Then later, when as a young adult I watched my stepmother die of complications from rheumatoid arthritis, I almost expected her death. I had unconsciously developed a belief that when people I loved became seriously ill they always got worse, never better.

Now, many years later, I wondered how I could release those hopeless fears and beliefs that had built up inside until they were being expressed in my own illness. Where was I going to find the hope and trust I needed to deal with what was happening to me?

The poet Ramakrishna wrote long ago, "The winds of grace blow all the time. All we need to do is to set our sails." Even though I felt unsure about how to begin ridding myself of fear and judgment about my body, I set my sails. I knew somehow that if it were something I truly wanted, ways to get there would come into my life.

Since then I've been amazed by the many opportunities that have come my way, that have allowed me to shift my feelings about my body from fear to appreciation. As I have embraced them, they have brought about a gradual but monumental shift from believing my body to be something negative, to trusting in the grace of its innate strength and ability to heal.

One significant opportunity arose when I discussed my confusion about how to rid myself of this debilitating body fear with Deborah Singleton, Director of a center called A Healing Place. Deborah has the ability to go to the core of significant concepts and describe them in terms that people can understand. She explained to me that my unhealthy beliefs and emotions generate certain frequencies in my body. These frequencies are the mind-body connection in action. When I move into more trusting beliefs, the frequencies change for the better. She talked to me about my body fear and suggested an exercise that over time has helped me change fear into trust:

------ ⌘ ------

I find a place to settle where I won't be interrupted. I give myself plenty of time and slowly ease into a deep and comfortable breathing rhythm.

I conjure up all the things I fear that might happen to my body. I imagine the worst: being crippled, destitute, full of unremitting pain, wasting away and even dying from arthritis. As my thoughts keep coming, I ride the wave of emotion until slowly, after two or three minutes, I feel the intensity dissipate.

I remind myself to maintain an easy breathing rhythm. Then I go back in my mind to a time or experience when my body felt strong and healthy. I let myself feel truly good in my body, and hold the sensation right now in this moment. I feel my hands tingle and wiggle my toes. I sink into my breathing and feel the rhythm of my chest rising and falling. I take time to relish this feeling.

I think about something positive that will replace my body fear. I focus on my body's innate strength and resilience, its healing intelligence. I remind myself that I don't know the exact answers, but I will work with my body to help it move toward health. Again, I take time to be with those good feelings.

I ask for help to release my body fear. As I ask for guidance from my spirit, relief washes over me, as if the heavy wave of emotion I have been riding has become a calm pool of water. I feel safe.

Finally, I picture myself with light flooding my whole body. I visualize my feet firm on the earth, as if I am a great oak tree with deep abiding roots. I feel stable and balanced.

This uplifting exercise has been an effective tool to help rid me of my old baggage of body fear. It doesn't happen overnight; the fear dissolves slowly, layer-by-layer. Often I'm not even aware that another layer of my fear is gone until I react positively to something that in the past would have thrown me into fear's grip.

Not long ago I wrote a farewell letter to my body fear. Getting my thoughts and feelings down on paper was another strong step forward.

Dear Body Fear,

You've been with me a long time. You are so familiar that I tend to believe everything you say must be true, especially when you remind me of things that I could have done and didn't, or start me worrying about what may happen in the future.

All these worries keep me from enjoying the present moment, and block my body from becoming healthier. Your unwelcome company affects how my body works. My breath changes and becomes shallow, closing the gates of energy that feed my cells. My stomach tightens and restricts the natural absorption of food. My heart feels your presence and reacts in primal ways.

I not only feel you in my body, but also in my mind. A favorite theme of yours is that anything negative that happens is bound to get worse. A health problem is a fruitful area for you, a place where all sorts of imaginary worst case scenarios fester—from a new small pain that might lead to something dangerous, to ominous blood test results.

A particularly troublesome belief you whisper to me when I'm not feeling well is that my health issues are somehow entirely my fault. I must have done something wrong.

I'm putting you on notice that I am stopping this self-defeating thinking, because it always results in taking me down the slope of guilt and negative physical repercussions. I'm going to talk back to you in healthy, life affirming ways. I want to change some things you bring to my attention that hinder my feeling better, but I will not allow finger pointing. Your power to make me feel bad about myself will no longer go unchecked.

I must admit that I'm learning much from you, Body Fear. I understand that when I allow you to control me, I'm diminished. I'm making a conscious choice to stretch myself and look for positive solutions to situations that involve my health. I'm learning not to get mired in self-blame or expectations of the poorest outcome. I will live in the present and step out of your shadow.

Now that I see you more clearly and know what I can do to change, you are shrinking in power. I'm freeing myself from our abusive relationship. Your diminished strength brings new creativity to my life, room for more pleasure and trust.

And believe it or not, Body Fear, I do appreciate you. Without you I would never have experienced my innate strengths so clearly. I would never have learned so well that I can really trust my body.

As I build new and more positive beliefs, I reinforce them by reminding myself of situations and experiences when I had more strength and agility. I often bring up those memories, not to feel a yearning for the good old days, but as a reminder that my body knows what health is, and that it is resilient and ever-changing. As I let go of body fear and other old unwanted beliefs and emotions, I find new energy and health. It is a slow but very powerful process, like a large ship that turns in a new direction, moving surely toward a better destination.

The power we have to change our attitudes is much greater than we realize. The same is true of our bodies, which are in a constant regenerative process. Deepak Chopra, in his series, *Magical Mind, Magical Body,* describes our bodies as rivers of energy and information. At a fundamental level they want to move toward our highest good. It's easy to place boulders and impediments that block these rivers of health. It's much more challenging to positively align our minds, emotions, and spirits, and allow ourselves to float downstream toward healing.

To help you get a sense of your own body fear, try this:

———∞∞———

Take some time to consider what fears you have about your body. Write them down if you wish. On balance, do you see your body as something to fear? Does the uncertainty of what's going to happen to you in the future leave you feeling helpless and scared?

Now consider the words you use to describe certain areas of your body, especially those particularly affected by your illness. Do you find yourself talking about "my bad back" or "my weak stomach?" Do these words contain clues to your true feelings about your body?

Finally, try Deborah Singleton's exercise for building trust which I described earlier in this chapter, and see if some of those negative feelings begin to fade.

———∞∞———

All of these things—exercises, letters to our fears, focused introspection—are effective tools to help us understand and neutralize our negative attitudes toward our bodies. None of them, however, are magical cures that work instantly, because our body attitudes are deeply ingrained. But with diligent work, these attitudes will fade. That's important, because it's only when they fade and vanish that we can move forward into positive relationships with our bodies.

CHAPTER 3

Listening

> "I am learning to hold the shifting currents of my body—the subtle changes in temperature, muscle tension, thought, and mood—the way a sailor rides the wind by reading the ripples on the water."
>
> KAT DUFF, *THE ALCHEMY OF ILLNESS*

*A*ddressing *my negative attitudes was important, but I realized it wasn't enough. Although I'd moved into a more neutral place, I still treated my body as an object, like a car or an appliance. If I were going to work with it in any meaningful way, my body and I needed to work together. We had to communicate with each other. We needed a relationship.*

I am surprised over and over by the power of purpose, by the fact that when we sincerely change our intent, we can quickly alter things in major ways. Almost as soon as I decided that we needed to establish a mutually supportive relationship, I began to sense that my body had consciousness. Instead of "it," I began to think about my body as "she."

Discovering that my body is in some ways not just a machine but almost like another person was at first fairly anxiety producing. What if I didn't like her? I couldn't just decide not to hang out with her. Do I blame her for being inadequate, allowing me to become ill? I had enough challenges just taking care of myself. Was I ready to take on the most intimate of dependents? Who is she?

Over time I have come back to the middle, cut back a bit on the anthropomorphizing. My body isn't a separate woman, she's my body—a part of me. She does have consciousness, though, and emotions lodge deeply in her flesh. Most importantly, she usually tries to do what's best for both of us, and she isn't a stranger. My body is like an old dear friend, and she and I are inseparable. I had arrived in and would leave from this same body. She had not abandoned me; it was more that I had abandoned her.

I remember coming across a workbook containing beautiful drawings of human anatomy and the interrelationship of its parts— muscles, tendons, joints, and organs all intertwined and working together. I was amazed at their complexity and inter-connectedness. The workbook helped me to see my body as something precious, a worthy companion to listen to and appreciate. It brought home to me the fact that when I ignore and distance myself from my body, I cut off a vital part of myself, the house of my spirit.

Next came a fairly difficult step for someone who had held her body at arm's length for so long. In order to reconnect, I needed to reach deeper into her, develop a more vital connection, really feel what was going on inside. I had to move from knowing intellectually that my body is complex and interesting, to experiencing her intimately.

It was hard to bring myself to open that door and actually step across the threshold. I was coming from a great distance, a lifetime of distrust and belief that bodies are betrayers and untrustworthy. It's something I've had to work at over the long haul.

I'm getting better at it, at quieting myself to feel and listen to all that is going on within me. I enjoy putting my hand on my heart and sensing the steady rhythm. It's invigorating to focus my attention on my hands and feet, and feel them tingle.

My body is a very busy and responsive creature. Something creative happens when I visualize my organs operating seamlessly, imagine my blood flowing and my connective tissue becoming more pliable. I picture nutrients filling me with strength and waste leaving. I often place a comforting hand on an area that is tight or hurts, and feel its response. The time I consciously spend with my body is something from which we both benefit, a connection that we've been yearning for all these years.

My determination to connect with my body led me to search for a type of exercise that would help me move deeper. Near my home was a tai chi center, and I stopped in to see what tai chi was like. I watched a class and was intrigued by the gracefulness and skill of this ancient Chinese movement system, and I thought about signing up for a beginning group.

As I was considering whether or not to join the class, my mind automatically dredged up the tired discouraging messages, the old litany of reasons why I shouldn't risk trying new things. It was telling me that tai chi was beyond my capability, dangerous, something that would probably stretch me too far.

I recognized the messages as the old limiting thoughts they were, but it's hard sometimes to know when to expand beyond our comfort level. One method I've found useful for making this kind of decision is to play a game that bypasses my mind and helps me intuitively discover whether a particular course of action is one I want to follow.

I visualize myself sitting in a theater with a large movie screen in front of me. I relax, sit back, and watch the action. In this case, I saw myself doing tai chi. As I watched myself, I focused on what I was feeling. Did it feel energizing, something I wanted to do? Or did the whole idea feel draining; something that I didn't really want to get involved with? I've found that this is a good way to listen to what my body and spirit need. My intuitive response to the tai chi movie in my mind was an easy, uplifting "yes."

Over the months that followed, I struggled at times with the rigors of tai chi, but for the most part I enjoyed what I was doing and discovered that I was regaining agility and confidence that I hadn't thought possible. I rid myself of an awkward walking gait. My body felt looser and more relaxed. Most importantly, while doing tai chi, I felt my mind and body in harmony.

When I moved to New Mexico many years later, I couldn't make myself practice tai chi. There was no tai chi group available and I had more pain and stiffness in my shoulder that made the moves difficult. When I didn't do the exercise, though, it left me feeling guilty that I wasn't continuing an activity that had been so useful and affirming.

In some ways I had come full circle—I again dreaded doing exercise. This time, however, I decided to respond differently. Instead of just criticizing myself, I looked for something new that would fit my needs. I discovered a DVD that demonstrated nei gong, a system of gentle stretching movements that emphasized releasing tension in the body. Nei gong was not only about slow movement but also involved deep breathing and releasing pent-up energy that holds patterns of stress. I found a local nei gong teacher and learned the form. I still do nei gong, and will continue until my body and my spirit tell me, through my inner voice, that it no longer meets my needs.

I'm finally beginning to trust my body. I've learned that understanding what I'm doing isn't as important as listening to what I'm feeling while I'm doing it. My body wants to feel trusted, to be allowed to flow with movement, all without criticism.

Whether we listen or not, our bodies are constantly trying to communicate with us. An especially familiar message from my body is "I'm feeling tired and worn out." Like many of us who were taught that we should get our work done before we relax, my old unconscious response was to ignore the message. I would automatically push on until I finished whatever I was doing, and often pay the price in stiffness and exhaustion.

Since I've started to listen, when I feel weariness in the midst of an activity, I ask myself, "Should I finish what I'm doing right now or take a rest?" Then if I can (sometimes you just have to push on), I give myself permission to rest.

I finally understand that there will always be more tasks to do. When I give myself time to nap or sit quietly, I affirm that one of the most important tasks on my to-do list is to take good care of myself.

In addition to forcing myself to keep going, I used to eat or drink things with caffeine, sugar, or preferably both, even though I knew I would feel more tired a few hours later. Now I do a better job of listening to my body's needs, and more often choose sustaining ways of gaining energy, such as drinking a glass of water, stopping what I'm doing to take deep breaths, and taking whatever time I need to rest.

Food is an area where even though our bodies have strong opinions, we tend to ignore them. We are continuously making decisions about food and getting feedback from our bodies in the form of how the food makes us feel. In my case, I've learned over time, for instance, that when I eat too many foods with refined sugar and wheat I will quickly feel lower energy, have stiffer joints, and perhaps experience a headache.

Guilt is another thing that can hold us in old, unhealthy patterns. Throughout our lives we've all been taught that exercising, getting plenty of rest, and eating right are important to health, and we know it's true. We know what the standards are and we know when we stray from them, so we carry around a lump of guilt because we aren't taking adequate care of ourselves. Ironically it's often the guilt itself that most hinders our ability to live better. Guilt can be a short-term motivator, but a barrier to making healthy long-term lifestyle shifts.

Even when we do things that are good for us, guilt can erode the value of the benefits. If I exercise, for instance, responding to the full chorus of "shoulds," the "shoulds" will keep me from listening to my body about whether the exercise is really good for me. If I stop and take a break when I'm worn out, but feel guilty because my "shoulds" tell me I should be pushing on, the value of the rest will be less because I'll still be tense. If I eat healthy food not because I'm listening to my body but because my critical voice demands it, my craving for unhealthy foods increases.

On the other hand, I've noticed there is a momentum and synergy that occur when I start making healthier choices because I want to, not because I'm responding to guilt. I want mindful exercising in my life because it makes me feel better and leads me to want healthier foods. I want to rest and slow down, not because I should but because it gives me more energy for the remainder of the day.

At first, I had to go on blind trust that all this effort was worthwhile. When I tried to exercise more or eat better, my mind would tell me that these small daily changes wouldn't make any real difference. As I kept feeling the good results of improving my daily habits, though, I no longer had to pretend I was getting better. I really was, and that in turn motivated me to continue and expand my healthier lifestyle.

We make a succession of decisions throughout each day, many unconsciously. If we can adopt the intent to be more aware when we make decisions that affect our well-being, we will gradually make them better. As we do this, even our unconscious decisions will improve.

One area where we obviously don't make a decision is whether to breathe or not, but we do have choices about how we breathe. We can use our breath to manage our minds, and it's an especially effective way to directly communicate with our bodies, asking them to relax and revitalize.

We breathe approximately 20,000 times a day. Each breath we take is an opportunity to unburden our minds from incessant chatter, let go of stress, and center ourselves.

Some time ago I came across a simple breathing exercise developed by Andrew Weil, M.D., that he calls Conscious Breathing. I use it often, because it helps me utilize my breath for my own healing.

I begin by placing my tongue just behind my teeth on the roof of my mouth. I quietly inhale through my nose, and exhale noisily through my mouth. The sound I make when I exhale is a kind of whoosh.

I inhale again through my nose to a count of four, hold my breath to a count of seven, and exhale through my mouth to a count of eight. As I exhale through my mouth, I try to rid myself completely of all the air in my lungs.

When I began doing this exercise, I repeated my breathing cycle four times. I did this several times a day. As I got used to it, I increased the number of cycles. At first, I sometimes felt light-headed. It took some time to get used to the increased oxygen.

Once I had practiced this four-seven-eight rhythm for awhile, I no longer needed to keep track by counting. It came naturally as I simply followed my breath with my mind, and experienced the expanded energy and peace that followed.

I now use my breath exercise almost without thinking, whenever I want to calm myself down, raise my energy, or diminish pain.

Merely becoming aware of our breath is a powerful way to center ourselves. Try focusing on your own breathing during activities that make you impatient, such as standing in a long line or hurrying because you're late for an appointment. It's a simple way to slow yourself down and relax, no matter what's happening.

Tuning in to our breath gives us insight into what's going on within us. Shallow breathing, for instance, is sometimes an indication of physical or emotional discomfort. By consciously slowing and deepening our breath, we enable ourselves to relax in the midst of stress or pain. Breathing straight into discomfort helps ease it.

Using our breath this way is not an act of collapsing into discomfort but of accepting it, removing some of its power. When we breathe directly into pain or anxiety and exhale restriction with our breath, we give ourselves relief and freedom.

Most profoundly, breath is an avenue for consciously developing a deeper connection with our spirit. People have been aware of the link between breath and spirit for centuries. The Sanskrit term for soul, *atman*, means both breath and life. A Hebrew word, *ruach*, means soul, wind or breath.

Our breath is a wonderful tool for turning our attention away from the outside world's frenetic calling. It brings us back home into our spirit. It's amazing the power that a single conscious breath has to return us into the center of ourselves.

When we work diligently on our relationship with our bodies, the relationship eventually becomes part of our habitual life. We don't have to think about checking in with our bodies when we make decisions; it happens automatically. We relax as our integration becomes an unconscious process, and we can be startled when some event reminds us just how far we have advanced.

A few years ago, my physician told me that a routine blood test had uncovered the fact that my blood sugar was very high, and that I had diabetes. Because he wanted to make it clear that there was no question about my condition, he firmly stated that I didn't have a borderline or pre-diabetic condition, but full-blown diabetes. He told me I didn't need to inject insulin now but my condition could worsen over time, and I might eventually need daily insulin shots.

He referred me to a nutritionist to begin learning how to balance carbohydrates and proteins, gave me a prescription for a blood testing device, and sent me out the door.

This was one of those "ton of bricks" situations. I had no symptoms pointing to diabetes, and none of my previous blood tests had even hinted that I had the disease. I walked into my doctor's office feeling fairly good, and walked out with a diagnosis of another life-long challenge.

If I'd been hit with this diagnosis earlier in my life, it would have left me awash with helplessness and fear. I would have instantly felt separated from the people around me. But this time, it didn't happen—in fact, when I checked with my body, it didn't even feel as if I had diabetes. I knew, though, that if I did have it, my body and I would manage it together. I surprised myself by thinking, "She and I can deal with this problem."

I got my blood monitor and met with the nutritionist. During the following months I monitored my blood sugar, controlled my food, and increased my exercise with more walking (something I wanted to do anyway). I did what I needed to do medically, and allowed very little space in my life for anxiety.

At my next check-up, my physician was very surprised to see that my blood sugar had returned to normal. The only explanation he could conceive of was that the high blood sugar indicated by the first test was caused by a medication I was taking. My blood tests have continued to confirm that I don't have diabetes. I never did tell my doctor that I was pretty sure all along that I didn't have the disease.

My work toward reducing my body fear had paid what seemed to me to be spectacular dividends. I hadn't responded to the diagnosis of diabetes with helplessness and fear as I would have earlier, but with the knowledge that my body was my friend, and the two of us could move through this together.

That experience was my own secret victory. My doctor, my family, and my friends never knew how I'd reacted that day when I was given my diagnosis, but I did. It was a wonderful indication to me of the distance I had come in dealing with fear and establishing a relationship with my body. On occasion, what seems at the time like a terrible event can carry a surprising gift.

When we desire a meaningful relationship with our bodies, we begin an ever-evolving movement toward strength and wholeness. As with any significant shifting, the process brings a mixture of ups and downs, confusions and insights. One thing, though, is for sure. When we decide to truly appreciate our body, feel its vitality and listen to its wisdom, we become abiding partners in our own healing.

CHAPTER 4

Moving From Roles to Real

"Sometimes I go about pitying myself. And all the while I am being carried on great winds across the sky."

TRADITIONAL OJIBWAY SAYING

*W*hen I received an announcement of a weekend seminar in Dallas, I was surprised at my eagerness to attend. It was one of those things that seem to drop into your lap at just the right time. I don't know why it grabbed my attention, but I suddenly decided to go. Normally, because of my physical limitations, I wouldn't have dreamed of doing something like that. The trip would involve driving five hundred miles from Kansas City to Dallas, which seemed as impossible as driving to the other side of the world.

In addition to the physical challenges, there were all sorts of unknowns. I'd be going by myself and although I had met the teacher a few months earlier, I wouldn't know any of the other participants. The workshop was occurring in a rural area outside of Dallas that would be difficult to find. I asked a good friend to go with me, but at the last minute there was an emergency that kept her home. Despite the grave doubts that swirled around me and knowing that I'd have to stop at least every hour to unlock my painful joints, I felt an intense desire to attend, and I decided to go.

During the drive it seemed as if I stopped more than I moved, but eventually I got there. Years later, when I'd become much healthier *and stronger, someone who had been at the seminar said I was so thin that it looked like the wind could blow me away.*

That weekend opened me up to a new world of awareness. It seemed as if the seminar leader were talking directly to me as she described how each person must find his or her own spiritual path. She emphasized that often the search begins in earnest when we are humbled by our most difficult life situations and thrust into unknown territory. Our experiences may give us a gentle nudge or, as in my case, a hard push. Rheumatoid arthritis had shaken me to my very roots.

She went on to say that true self-discovery is not about searching for answers "out there," but about finding wisdom within. Our inner wisdom is based on a fundamental truth that our spirit is the heart of our identity. On the surface, our earthly identities make us seem widely different from each other. But when we shed our external differences—things like our occupations, personal stories, and our own mixture of beliefs and habits—we discover that we share a common spiritual essence.

As I sat listening, I had a strong sense that I was not alone. My external identity may have dramatically changed when I became ill, but heightened awareness of my spirit's unchanging presence was becoming stronger. I realized that at my core, I was essentially the same person I had always been. I understood that my spirit had always been present within me, waiting to lead the way in my life.

After the seminar was over, I started for home feeling much lighter. My spirit was lifting me up. At one point I remember a few drivers passing my car, and feeling love flow toward them. In those moments, I had a growing awareness that I was connected to everything, even strangers on the interstate.

Shortly after returning from Dallas, I happened to pick up a book by Louise Hay called, *You Can Heal Your Life,* in which she describes how different diseases can be manifestations of our fundamental emotional patterns. As I thumbed through her book and all the maladies she discussed, I came to rheumatoid arthritis and saw the words "feeling very put-upon."

The phrase irritated me, which was a sure sign that it had hit home. I instantly thought, "That isn't me." In fact, because I didn't have any real understanding of the strong link between my body and my mind and emotions, I doubted that my struggles could be at all related to non-physical issues. As I became weaker and in more pain, however, it began to dawn on me that my body was trying to teach me something. I thought about Louise Hay's book, and about what it means to feel "very put-upon."

I realized that my self-esteem was based to a great extent on my need to be needed. I'd even picked a career in counseling, a profession that extended my being helpful beyond family and friends to a wider circle of people. Helpful sounds like a good way to be, but I began to realize that in my case I'd been draining myself dry.

Over the years, I had internalized the belief that it was selfish to focus on myself and that others should always come first. I thought if I were a good helper I would get some support in return, but it never occurred to me that healthy support starts within myself. I now realize how very difficult it was for others to understand my needs, when I didn't even know what they were myself.

My way of taking care of people was to absorb their problems, which was a huge drain on my energy. It was not only unhealthy for me, but it took from others their right to manage their own struggles. I now know that I stayed involved with everyone else in part so that I didn't have to look inside.

In those days, I had all sorts of insights and opinions about what others should be doing. When people didn't follow my advice I would feel anger, but I held my frustration in check because it didn't correspond with my self-image.

If I had looked inside, I would have discovered that my anger wasn't at the other person at all; it was really at myself for my own imbalance. I resented that I had adopted a job description that never changed: "Be a person who needs to be needed and resists taking care of herself."

When I finally looked honestly I saw how I felt "very put-upon," and the rocks of resentment I was piling on my own back were getting heavier and heavier. Resentment was part of the reason arthritis moved so vigorously within me, and it was certainly contributing to my growing weakness. My suppressed feelings of frustration toward others and myself had found a hidden home.

In our area of rural New Mexico, there are rattlesnakes that come near our garden wall and sometimes right into the yard. I find them scary but also fascinating. My heart always skips a beat when I hear the clicking of their rattles and see their heads raised and bobbing, as they protect themselves from unknown danger. Once in a while I find a tattered ribbon of old skin shed by a snake during its yearly ritual, brittle and dull brown and useless.

A snake shedding its skin is not so different from what I was going through as I worked to release the rigid roles I had automatically assumed as wife, mother, daughter, sister, counselor, and friend. I was becoming aware of how those roles defined and ladened me with heavy self-expectations that hindered honest relationships with others, and that interfered with having an authentic relationship with myself. Merely becoming conscious of those burdens was the start of shedding old restrictive roles.

This became particularly clear to me through an experience I had with my father.

In the last years of his life, my father began losing some of his independence due to a mild stroke and problems with his eyes. It became apparent that I needed to start paying his bills and taking care of other business matters for him.

Once I assumed this role, I noticed that our enjoyable conversations and the good feelings we'd always shared were fading. He became distracted and agitated whenever I started writing checks and doing other business tasks for him. To be truthful, I was irritated that he didn't seem to appreciate what I was doing.

One day it occurred to me that I was rushing into his apartment focused on getting things done, when all we both really wanted was to visit and enjoy our time together as we had in the past. Most of our earlier visits had been spent reminiscing about old times, enjoying good laughs, and watching the birds outside his window. My visits were now highlighting for him his loss of independence, and for me frustration over losing the loving connection of our old relationship. I knew I needed to change something—my visits were very significant to him, especially as he had fewer visitors and outside contacts in his last few years of life.

I decided to change my attitude and approach. First, I changed the way I took care of his business matters. My visits began with looking at what had to get done and ways to proceed, and I would take the paperwork home to do later. Then we would put business aside and just enjoy our time together.

His apartment was on the second floor, and I used the short ride in the elevator to slow my pace and calm down. In those few moments I could feel the hassles of traffic and the hectic pace of my day slip away. By the time I knocked on his door I was ready to enjoy our visit, which as I look back after his death, was some of the most precious time we had.

I went a step further, and made a habit of regularly checking with myself to see whether my visits were motivated by truly wanting to go, or by feelings that I should go. I made a bargain with myself that if "shoulds" were the only thing pressuring me to go see my dad I'd wait, if at all possible, until it was something I actually wanted to do. Surprisingly, when I calmed myself down and observed my feelings of guilt and obligation, they seemed to fade away.

Sometimes when I was feeling overburdened, I used an exercise that helped me release those unwanted feelings. I continue to use it today for letting go of immediate frustration and resistance.

I close my eyes and connect with my body by taking deep slow breaths. I visualize a band of white light circling clockwise around me. I allow myself to feel the spinning circle of light.

Next, I imagine reversing the band of light so it rotates around me in the opposite direction, counter-clockwise. Once the light is turning easily, I gently push my agitation and worry into the band, which flings it out and away.

I stay with this a few minutes, gently breathing, until my negativity is gone. Then I bring my band of light back into a comforting clockwise circle around me, and sink into its ease.

What a simple discernment, to feel the difference between being driven by obligation and being motivated by truly wanting to do something. What a revelation it was when I saw that attending to my own needs carried benefits for others as well.

People define themselves in many ways. "Who are you?" is a difficult question for most of us, because there are many levels at which we could respond. Our first response might be to describe ourselves based on the work we do. It's easy to define ourselves as a teacher or a lawyer or salesperson, but what happens when we lose our job or retire or have to stop working? What if we retain our job, but it no longer has meaning for us? Then who are we?

Others might describe themselves primarily in terms of their relationships—their marriage or their roles as parent, sister, or son. Defining ourselves by our relationships carries the same risk as defining ourselves by our occupation, because they both leave little room for an expanded view of who we are, and they both put us in a vulnerable position. If our relationships become problematic or terminate, it's all too easy to feel like a failure as a person.

Dawna Markova, in her book, *I will not Die an Unlived Life: Reclaiming Purpose and Passion*, expresses all this beautifully:

> We become accustomed to identifying ourselves as nouns, as small, enclosed, exclusive, and local units: friend, artist, mother. It's as if we spend so much time close to the canvas carefully painting tiny purple dots in a Pointillist painting, that we have forgotten how to step back enough to get a sense of the whole.
>
> Yet it is only from this perspective that we can learn to see the overall pattern that we have been creating, the verbs we have been living—creating, befriending, mothering—which are the horizons we need to move toward.

Sometimes we define ourselves by our situation or experiences. As I discussed earlier, with the onset of a disease, for instance, we may define ourselves primarily as a sick person. We reinforce this new identity with almost constant activities that focus on our illness: going to doctors, obsessing about our health problems, and talking about how we feel to the exclusion of other subjects.

Often, as in my advanced case of "service to others," our concept of who we are comes from experiences in our early environment, when we watched and emulated how people important to us defined themselves, and what they expected from us.

A client of mine who suffered from chronic fatigue told me that when he was growing up, everyone in his family had to be productive and stay busy. As a child, if his mom saw him playing, watching television, or reading a book, she would call him "lazy bones" and give him a task to do. He learned that to be of value, he always had to be doing something productive.

In later years, when confronted with severe physical problems that required a great deal of rest, his mother's critical voice was still running in his head, calling him lazy and demanding that he get up and do something useful. It's all too easy for other people's judgments and expectations to become what we think we are supposed to be.

When Marc, an old friend, was confronted with fibromyalgia, he made a wonderful shift away from his old voices. He was able to go beyond the restraints of his illness and banish most of the old expectations he had absorbed, and discover and honor who he really was at his core.

Over the span of his interesting life Marc had various careers, and in his later years he became a small business consultant. He enjoyed helping people develop plans that would transform their passionate ideas into concrete actions. But when he started experiencing muscle pain and extreme lack of energy, Marc could no longer function as he had in the job he loved.

At first, he thought he would have to give up his business completely. After a period of time, however, he realized that he could apply his teachings to his own situation, so Marc created a plan for himself, as he'd done for so many others. He called it his life plan and it included a much slower-paced lifestyle, plenty of quiet contemplative time, and regular exercise at a nearby rehabilitation center. He and his wife honored their desire to serve by making monthly meals they delivered to people who were homeless, and he even kept his consulting business on a more limited basis.

More importantly, Marc's shift brought benefits that went way beyond his work, his relationships, and his activities. Because he'd altered his life in ways that nurtured his spirit, there was a new sparkle in his eyes and an apparent contentment. Even though he felt severe discomfort at times, he didn't let his illness define him. What shone brightly was his new connection to his spirit.

Shakti Gawain in her book, *The Path of Transformation,* discusses what it means when our spiritual nature leads us:

> Contact with our spiritual self gives us an expanded perspective on our lives, both as individuals and as part of humanity. Rather than just being caught up in the daily frustration and struggles of our personality, we are able to see things from the perspective of the soul. We are able to look at the bigger picture of life on earth, which helps to understand a lot more about why we're here and what we're doing. It helps to make our daily problems seem not so huge and makes our lives more meaningful.

When I think back on how I headed for that seminar in Dallas despite feeling sick and scared, I realize that my spirit was beginning to come forward. Somehow I had started to trust my unknown journey. I was beginning to get a glimmer of what I understand now: Wherever life takes me, it's my spirit I will trust.

CHAPTER 5

Hearing the Voices

"The voice in the head has a life of its own.
Most people are at the mercy of that voice;
they are possessed by thought, by the mind."

ECKHART TOLLE, *A NEW EARTH*

*O*ne day on a hike with friends in search of
a remote waterfall, my weary body stepped down on a rock that was
much lower than I expected. Immediately I felt a fierce pain in my
knee. "Oh boy," I thought, "I'm in deep trouble."

*Earlier a small voice inside my head had suggested I take a rest
and let my companions keep on exploring without me, but I wouldn't
listen to it. My determination to keep up and find the waterfall
drowned out my quiet voice. That one misstep triggered a flare-up
throughout my body, from which it took months to recover.*

After I hurt my knee, it didn't take long for my inner critic to
come alive. It's the strident voice we all have, that only speaks words
of self-judgments and negativity. My critic chided me for taking such
a vigorous hike. It told me I should have known better, that what I
had done was a really dumb thing. It ominously assured me that this
was the start of a downhill spiral that would only get worse. One of
the most debilitating aspects of the inner critic is that it speaks with
such authority and certainty.

As I was recovering from my flair-up in the months that followed,
I realized that I had allowed this toxic thinking to gain momentum
and dominate my perspective toward myself. It was as if the voice

were muttering constantly in the background, a grinding and grating noise. It spoke familiar helpless refrains of "I can't," "I must," "if only." I realized that as I listened to those words over and over again, they became a self-fulfilling prophecy that made me lose ground. Those poisonous messages were doing real damage.

I decided that the first thing I had to do to free myself of that debilitating voice was to create a space so I could separate from all its negative commotion. I went on alert so I could catch the voice as it came to the fore, and then try to tone it down, push it away, maybe even turn it off.

Once I had a little breathing space, I worked to develop an understanding of just how the critical voice operated. Not surprisingly, I learned that I was more vulnerable to those negative mantras when I was feeling insecure and unsure of myself, such as when I was depressed or in pain. I began to observe the voice in those vulnerable moments, and consciously replace its harping with positive thoughts. One technique that was especially useful was to ask myself, "What can I do right now to feel better?" I replaced negative thoughts with a mental search for a positive action.

I found that as my negative voice faded, a consistently supportive voice developed. I called the new voice "the observer" because it spoke affirmatively with gentle authority, like a caring friend who could look at my situation from an analytical distance. My observer voice gives me positive guidance and helpful perspectives.

At first, it took me awhile to get used to this voice. I was surprised to find encouraging thoughts coming forward when I was feeling bad. In the past, I would have had to go to a trusted friend or my husband to find a positive voice. Now I'm more able to generate and call upon my own supportive and hopeful thoughts.

I particularly remember one time when my inner critic was harping at me, and my observer voice whispered, "Wouldn't it make sense for you to be most loving to yourself when you hurt and need help?"

That was the fundamental change I was working toward, and feeling it expressed so clearly inside helped me step firmly away from the fading nag of my critical voice.

My emerging observer voice has a caring quality that is decidedly different from my critical one. It's not based on negativity and blaming, but on common sense and a broader view of my situation. When I'm discouraged, my observer voice reminds me that nothing is permanent and says such things as, "How you feel right now will pass. You've made it through hard times before, and you'll do it again." Every time I affirm positive words such as these, they become stronger and more believable and eventually come automatically. These bits of positive self-talk help move me into a place where instead of being blocked by "I can't," I'm carried forward by "I will."

In her book, *Molecules of Emotion*, scientist Candace Pert explains that the brain, glands, spleen, bone marrow, and lymph nodes are all linked together in a network of communication. She states that "The mind doesn't dominate the body, but is a part of the body—body and mind are one." She calls this network the bodymind.

Pert and other scientists have shown how our emotions trigger the release of chemicals throughout the body, which in turn alter the way we physically feel. In particular, the scientific data clearly demonstrate that chemicals generated by our thoughts and general attitudes reduce or increase our pain.

Our thoughts create emotions. When we allow thoughts from our inner critic to go unchecked, as I was doing after my hiking accident, they create negative emotions that drain our energy and vitality and make us feel physically worse. Although we are aware that we feel worse, we are usually unaware that it's in part because of our negative self-talk.

Our thoughts also directly affect our physical strength. This fact can be dramatically demonstrated by an exercise I did with a group of young teen-age girls at a time when I was doing school social work. A teacher asked me to come to her class because there was a problem with a small group of girls who were bullying others.

When I walked into the classroom, I could sense animosity and defensiveness from the bullying group. They knew why I was there and were naturally concerned about how I was going to deal with them. I casually introduced myself, and told the class we were going to do an exercise that might surprise them.

I asked Melanie, one of the girls in the troublesome clique, if she'd come to the front of the room to help me demonstrate something. I told her to hold her arm straight out at shoulder height and resist as I pulled her arm down, which I did without too much difficulty.

Next, while she held her arm out again, I asked her to close her eyes and think about an experience where she had felt really good about herself. She closed her eyes and by a slight smile on her face, we could all see that she was remembering something pleasant. This time when I tried to pull her arm down, Melanie had become surprisingly strong, and it took both my hands and a great deal of effort to finally bring her arm to her side.

Then I asked her to concentrate on a time when she had been embarrassed, or someone had said something that hurt her feelings. She held the same arm straight out once again, and this time I quickly pulled her arm down with almost no effort. Melanie opened her eyes and with a look of amazement asked, "What happened?"

There were doubtful glances among the other girls who had been watching, so I asked each girl to find a partner and try this same exercise. Interestingly, several of the girls who had been hurting others happened to team up with girls they'd bullied. Even after they'd gone through the exercise and had an experience similar to Melanie's, a few still couldn't believe it. I suggested they repeat the exercise for a second time, which they did with the same results.

We discussed at length how thoughts and stinging words hurt and weaken our bodies. The old saying, "Sticks and stones can break my bones, but names can never hurt me," just isn't true. What we dwell on and how our inside voices talk to us have concrete consequences for our bodies, and it's good for all of us to pay attention to them and work to make them more positive.

Also, beneath the negative and positive voices there is yet another voice, one that we all have, a "wee small voice" that emanates from our spirit. It's an intuition that comes from our inner vision and slips quietly into our minds. It can be a soft insight, a knowing without factual basis, or a sense that something is just right or wrong. Because it seems to come out of the blue, we label it as intuition.

We all have intuition, and it often speaks to us through our feelings. It's a part of the legacy we brought with us when we were born into the world. Before we knew language, we relied on unfiltered sensing and feeling to alert us to what was happening around us. As we grew older, though, the direct experiences we had as babies had to change and adapt. We learned to rely mostly on learning and language, so we could navigate and resonate with the world and the people around us.

Part of my life's journey is to reclaim my intuition. I often visualize it as emanating from a presence watching from a balcony to the stage below, where I'm busily enmeshed in life's dramas. I think about the hard work my spirit undertakes as it slips through my mind's distracting noise and clatter, to offer what I need. I sometimes imagine myself on the stage, looking upward toward the balcony and asking for intuitive guidance. In unexpected ways and over time, I usually receive a response—an idea or direction, in one form or another. The messages can be as simple as reminding me to lighten up, or a gut feeling that something isn't right and I need to go in a different direction.

Intuition is a gift from our spirit. We don't have to change our thinking to benefit from it, as we do when we rid ourselves of our inner critic or when we employ our rational mind to think things through. In fact, it works best when we aren't thinking at all.

To reclaim and strengthen our intuition, all we need to do is open our hearts and listen. Over time, as we become quieter and more receptive, a gentle growing awareness will awaken the realization that our intuition is our spiritual birthright and that it has always been there for us.

Here's a way to become more familiar with your intuition:

The next time you are trying to make a hard decision, hold the issue close to you. Imagine it as a homing pigeon you are about to release. Ask yourself for direction toward your highest good. Picture releasing the pigeon and sending it deep within your spirit. See it spreading its wings to gather wisdom.

Over the next few days, watch for an answer. It may come in a dream, as a sudden insight, an off-hand remark by a friend, something you read or see, or in some other way. It may happen immediately or it may take longer, but when the time is right, your answer will find its way back to you.

CHAPTER 6

Transforming Dark Into Light

> "'Why,' she asked herself, 'why keep a wound
> open when forgiveness can close it?'"
>
> ALEXANDER MCCALL SMITH,
>
> *THE CUPBOARD OF LIFE*

*T*here was a hard knot in my stomach as I
ended the telephone call with my son who had phoned from 2,000 miles
away in Anchorage, Alaska. Our conversation had begun with catch-
ing up on what had been happening in our daily lives, then suddenly
jumped to the impact my divorce had had on him twenty years before.

This was a subject we had rarely discussed, so I was surprised
when he began expressing how difficult the divorce had been for
him as a young teen-ager. We'd never talked about those events in
such an honest and open way. It was obviously important for him,
so I encouraged him to share the strong feelings he had carried for
a long time. As we talked, my tightening stomach made me aware of
the strong feelings I still carried myself, after all those years.

Later, I thought about how helpful it had been for both of us. It
allowed him to get old issues off his chest, and it made me aware
that I had important work to do. I needed to rid myself of the guilt I
carried about my divorce. I had an image of myself as a donkey, bent
beneath a heavy load of emotions as I struggled up a steep incline. I
didn't want to carry that burden anymore.

I thought I had put my divorce to rest long ago, but Tim's call
showed me that painful feelings remained, raw and oppressive

beneath the surface. I still carried hurt and self-criticism from that period of my life, when my marriage failed and my illness began. I knew that I needed to be rid of those emotional burdens. I also knew the hardest part would be to forgive myself.

Most of us carry pain about hurtful events in our lives. It would be unusual if we didn't—life presents us with deep wounds, losses, and sadness, and they accumulate over time.

We also carry smaller wounds that may not be as deep, but still leave us hurt and diminished in some ways. They could come from many things: a moment when someone made us feel foolish, a situation where we didn't get what we thought we deserved, or a time when we were snubbed by a friend.

Whether we realize it or not, there is a part of us that wants to hold onto hard feelings. Maybe it's the part that needs to be right or the part that believes we're guilty and deserve the pain. Whatever its source, we often hang onto those feelings for a long time.

One might wonder why we should even bother with letting go of people or situations that have hurt us in the past, if we no longer think about them. But even though they may not be at the surface of our minds, the hurts are there, and they impact us in the present.

In Fred Luskin's book, *Forgive for Good,* he makes the point that grievances dramatically affect our health, because they keep alive the emotional and physical responses that accompanied the original experiences. He cites one study in which people who relived a hurtful situation and then imagined forgiving, had significantly lower blood pressure and heart rates than those who only relived the hurt. Our bodies hold on to difficult experiences, and we need to take conscious actions to diminish their effect on us.

Not only do old resentments affect our physical well-being, they also divert our attention and energy from enjoying the moment. Our tendency to hold on to those things is illustrated nicely by the story of two Zen monks who, while traveling, came across a young woman attempting to cross a muddy place on the road. It looked as if the woman would ruin her beautiful kimono, so one of the monks picked her up and carried her across.

After the monks had walked on silently for several hours, the one who had watched his companion carry the woman asked, "Why did you do that? You know we aren't supposed to do such a thing." The other monk smiled at his companion and answered, "I put the woman down hours ago. Why are you still carrying her?"

The resentments and guilt we accumulate over the years work together to sour our approach to life. We develop negative expectations. We begin to expect others to do us wrong and believe that upcoming situations will turn out badly. Our negative experiences spill over and darken our present, and seep into the future.

A habit that gives our difficult memories such intractable strength is that we often replay our painful stories the same way over and over in our minds, like broken records. Family and friends can also keep our grievance stories alive, as they develop and repeat their own versions. Those memories are like old familiar plays, and they almost always involve villains and victims.

Because the parts of villain and victim are laden with emotionally charged judgments of who was good and who was bad, they lock us into a single perspective about our memories. If we want to drain the strength from those old experiences, it's helpful to understand how the roles can change, depending on the outlook of different characters in the story.

We begin to release our old hurts and become more forgiving people when we're willing to look at our painful memories from all sides. We may be surprised, for instance, when we look through the eyes of the person we think of as a villain, to discover that he or she feels victimized themselves. They may carry their own burdens of hurt and guilt.

It's a challenge to look at all sides in a painful story, but we make significant headway when we open ourselves to others' views and emotions. We need to appreciate their fears, anxieties, and motivations if we want to unlock our memories and release the hurt we carry.

Another thing that was very helpful to me as I worked toward releasing my own grievance stories was to develop an understanding of the emotions that make them so powerful and resistant. Our grievances are usually fueled by two primary emotions, blame and guilt. They may seem like the opposite of each other, but at their core, blame and guilt are the same thing.

When we blame, we project our anger onto someone or something outside of ourselves. We see ourselves as victimized by someone else's actions and we often want revenge, but we usually find that getting even does not result in long-term emotional health or satisfaction. Revenge never leads to healing—it just reinforces our negativity.

As Nelson Mandela said, "Having resentment against someone is like drinking poison and then hoping it will kill your enemy." When we blame, we are the true losers. Even when we understand this, however, and decide we want to rid ourselves of old anger, we often experience a sense of helplessness, because blame gives someone else power over the events of the story—they "did it" to us. We may have to work hard to neutralize blame, because we have to assert control over events in which we have long seen ourselves as powerless.

With guilt, we point the finger at ourselves. As I looked at my own grievance story about my divorce, my feelings were mostly of guilt for not having been a good wife and mother. When I decided I didn't want to carry that guilt anymore, I was surprised at the strength of the resistance I encountered.

It dawned on me that despite the fact that those old remnants of guilt were damaging my health and sapping my energy, I resisted releasing them because I believed I deserved the punishment they inflicted. I needed to quit doing this, and the only way was to go into my story and try to truly understand it, so I could defuse the deep current of guilt it carried.

Whether our painful stories are based on blame or guilt, we have to do the same thing to take away their power: understand and forgive the villain. Before we can do that, we must understand the nature of our hurts and the forces that hold them tightly within us. It's difficult to forgive if we haven't built a foundation of understanding to support the process.

One good way to get a sense of the nature of the blame and guilt we carry about a particular event is to become an observer, to listen closely to ourselves as we think or talk about the story, and to notice how we feel. It's often the case that until we really observe ourselves, we aren't aware of how much we are stuck in the past.

A flash of resistance is an especially clear indicator of stuck anger or guilt. If we're discussing a painful event, for example, and someone casually mentions that perhaps the villain could be excused because of problems in their own life, do we immediately disagree? Does our stomach get tight and do our eyes narrow with denial? When a friend suggests that we shouldn't blame ourselves so much for a situation that turned out badly, do we feel a spasm of denial, a flush of shame?

Also, as we talk about what happened, where is our focus? Is it on guilt and blame, or on our emotions? There is a significant difference between talking about being angry at someone, and talking about being betrayed. When we talk about our anger, we at least acknowledge that we are responsible for our feelings and emotions. The emphasis is on how we feel, not on what was done to us. With feelings of betrayal, however, we are focusing on the actions of someone else, and our power over our emotions disappears in our role as victim.

Another aspect of listening to our old stories is to notice the people we talk to about what happened. Do we primarily revisit old painful experiences with people who reinforce how bad those experiences were, or do we seek out people who help us find new perspectives?

I was fortunate to have a friend who helped me get out of the rut of my divorce story by asking me the simple question, "What positive things are you willing to accept about that hard stage of your life?" I was so used to thinking about that difficult time in the old way that it took awhile to answer. When I did, I surprised myself by saying, "I really did the best I could. That was an important period of my life because it started me in a whole new positive direction." Her question moved me toward accepting what happened during that time without guilt or blame.

After my conversation with my son, I wrote him the following letter. It cleared away much for me, and it helped him as well.

Dear Tim,

I have thought often about our conversation a few months ago, when we talked about your dad's and my divorce, and the impact it had on you during your teenage years.

I know you felt that you lost both your parents during that time. We weren't able to give you adequate guidance in your turbulent years of adolescence, when parents are so needed. I didn't have room for opening my heart fully to you, so you could feel more cared for and supported.

I also didn't give you enough structure. I think I was afraid that if I disciplined more, the mother-son cord between us would be severed. These are not excuses; I know you must have felt as if I cut you too early from your moorings, left you adrift and wandering.

There is nothing I can do to make up for those years except to ask for your forgiveness and understanding. I want to release those sad times and free myself from self-criticism, and from continuing to think about what I might have done differently.

We have a deep and loving relationship, and I want the love I feel toward you to flow freely without guilt and remorse from the past. It's important for me to forgive myself, and to ask you, a person I love deeply, to forgive me as well. It allows me to feel free, open my heart, and appreciate our relationship and all that we both are.

One day after I sent the letter to Tim, I was going through a scrapbook, when I ran across an old photograph of me with my two young sons that was taken a few years before all the turmoil started. I looked closely at my smiling face. Did I have a clue then about what was going to happen in the near future? Did I know somewhere deep in the recesses of my psyche that my health was deteriorating, my marriage crumbling, and our lives were changing forever?

As those questions swirled through my mind, I felt a growing sense of respect for the person I became as I moved through all that difficulty. I knew that something that had been locked in darkness for a very long time was finally coming to light. Looking at the photograph flooded me with compassion for myself and for others who have been through similar times of pain and loss and growth.

Forgiveness opens our eyes, and allows us to see ourselves and our world very differently. It gives us space to learn from our mistakes. When we acknowledge our part in creating grievance stories and the drama that follows, we can take the next step and learn to avoid setting up such patterns in the future.

Some dear friends of mine had a son named Paul, who many years ago when he was twenty-one, was cycling in a triathlon. The highway route of the race was poorly marked and because Paul was leading, he was the first to reach an intersection where a semi-truck was coming through from the opposite direction. The truck struck Paul, and he was killed.

It was a terrible blow for those of us who knew and loved Paul, and his parents were devastated. Yet somehow in the midst of their grief, Paul's parents reached out to the truck driver and invited him into their home. They wanted the driver to know that they did not blame him for Paul's death, and they wanted to include him in the group of us who shared the pain.

I've always been amazed at their wisdom and ability to see the importance of that gesture, and grateful because it showed us that we're all connected. It raised us to a higher place and allowed Paul's parents and all who loved him to write our own stories of his death without the negative energy of blame.

When we rewrite our stories so that guilt and blame are diminished or removed, the memories become rich and alive. We free ourselves to understand how we've grown, and what we've learned. We don't deny our pain, but balance it with understanding of the power that adverse events can have to transform our lives.

It's not worth the price we pay to keep carrying our grievances. The longer we live with our resentments, the heavier our burdens become. Releasing guilt and blame opens us to spiritual wisdom and emotional resilience, and allows those qualities to continue to grow.

By forgiving ourselves and allowing blame and guilt to dissipate, we become more accepting and less judgmental. The process of letting go allows our difficult experiences to flow more easily through us and become positive rather than negative influences in our lives.

In tai chi, there is a martial art called push hands, where two people stand opposite each other with their wrists lightly touching. As the two people move back and forth, they look as if they're engaged in a graceful dance. Each person is probing for imbalance in the other.

A participant becomes vulnerable and is likely to fall when he or she pushes too vigorously or resists too directly the pushes of the opponent. The winner is the one who stays centered and balanced, delivering pushes without leaving his center, deflecting pushes so that his balance is maintained and the force passes ineffectively.

Push hands is a useful symbol for me. When an unwelcome experience is coming toward me, I think about letting it just go on by. If I find myself in a hurtful situation with the impulse to strike out, I think of push hands and remember to sink into my own strength and not get caught up in the anger of the moment.

When we strengthen our ability to forgive and accept, we find ourselves thinking less in terms of right and wrong, black and white. Instead of pointing our fingers, we open our eyes to see how we can understand and experience situations differently. By doing so, we gradually weaken destructive patterns. We move toward peace and away from drama. Above all else, we become more loving people.

Leonard Cohen, the great songwriter and poet, has a line in his song, "Anthem": "There is a crack in everything; that's how the light gets in." Forgiveness is a crack that lets love, growth, and peace into our lives.

Try this simple exercise:

The next time someone says something rude or hurtful to you, imagine their action as a wind blowing through you, leaving you untouched.

Breathe slowly and deeply into any knots and tensions, and feel them gradually ease and release.

When you return to the moment, notice how quieted and peaceful you are. Take a deep breath and center yourself in your balance.

CHAPTER 7

Finding Our Place in the World

"Following your bliss as Joseph (Campbell) meant it, is not self-indulgent but vital; your whole physical system knows that this is the way to be alive in this world and the way to give the world the very best that you have to offer. There is a track just waiting for each of us, and once on it, doors will open."

A JOSEPH CAMPBELL COMPANION
SELECTED AND EDITED BY DIANE K. OSBORN

I was sitting in a hotel room in Las Vegas with an infected right eye that had nearly swelled shut. The next morning I would present a workshop on "The Balancing Act--How to Balance Your Life." At that moment, however, I felt completely out of balance.

I was to give my program to a convention of meeting planners as an audition of sorts. Those who were attending would evaluate and choose the presenters they liked, so they could later hire them to make presentations at their own national meetings. I was in un-known territory and felt way out of my league.

I had started getting the eye infection on the flight to Las Vegas. With my face swollen and my eye almost closed, I wasn't in any shape to stand in front of an audience and present anything. I also had to deal with the problem of my arthritis, which was flaring up after the cramped quarters of a long flight and lugging my bags through two airports.

*In my hotel room many miles from home, I wondered how I had got-
ten myself into this mess. Accepting the invitation had seemed like such
a good idea at the time. I felt flattered that I had been invited, and didn't
ask myself the important question of whether this was something that
I really wanted to do. I probably wouldn't be giving my situation such
careful thought if I weren't experiencing this unusual problem with my
eye. It made me stop and think about what I wasn't seeing.*

*A few years before, I had interviewed with a national seminar
company that provided programming for women on self-esteem and
communication skills. The man who interviewed me talked about
going from city to city, setting up for the seminars in different hotels,
giving a number of six hour presentations, and selling books and
tapes about the subject. A day after my interview, I came down with
a flu from which it took me several weeks to recover. The recovery
time gave me an opportunity to realize that the national seminar job
was not a good fit for me.*

*Now my body was telling me the same thing again with the eye in-
fection. I was getting the clear message that what I was doing wasn't
good for me. When was I going to learn to honor these messages?*

*As I made my presentation the next day, I was exhausted.
Fortunately, my eye had started to recover so that I could at least
look out at the audience. The audio-visual equipment stopped work-
ing halfway through—one more indication that this scene wasn't for
me. Oddly though, once I realized that I wasn't meant to do this kind
of work, I felt calm despite the problems I encountered.*

*I couldn't wait to get out of town. The event had been a far cry
from what I had wished for. I realized that I wasn't going to be on
the top of any convention planner's list, but at a deeper level, I also
knew that I had finally begun to listen to my body's messages. As I
flew home, both my eyes were healthy and wide open.*

In the following months I thought a great deal about which activi-
ties give me energy and purpose, and which drain me. My Las Vegas

experience showed me one thing I didn't want to do, which was a good place to start.

Then something I really wanted to do popped up right in front of me. Not long after my trip, I was asked by our local Arthritis Foundation to lead a support group for young adults who have arthritis, and I accepted.

One of the most important things we did was to work toward finding and keeping meaning in our lives when physical challenges could easily steal it away. As we helped each other with sometimes big but often small problems, we learned significant lessons.

In the group, Edith was lamenting the fact that she could no longer handle the big family dinners she loved, because her hands were too sore to do the cooking. She had recently hosted a family gathering from which it took her several days to recover. Someone suggested that she make those gatherings potluck and spread the hosting responsibilities around. As she thought about it, Edith realized it wasn't making a fancy meal that was important to her, but having her family and friends gather together.

Edith's experience and those of others in our group helped us all appreciate how important it is to keep meaningful activities flourishing, modifying them if need be but preserving their essence.

We learned that new opportunities seem to multiply when we're committed to filling our lives with meaning. As Joseph Campbell, philosopher and teacher said, "I have found that you have only to take one step toward the gods and they then take ten steps toward you." A great example of this for us was an opportunity offered to our group by a regional arthritis center located in a large hospital in our community. The center asked me to write and host a video series on healthy living with arthritis, for other support groups to use.

The cooperative project represented a meaningful avenue to express my creativity. For our small arthritis group it was an opportunity to be involved and to share our experiences and the beliefs we had developed about healthy attitudes in dealing with chronic illness. After the project, we discussed its effect on us and agreed that it clarified what we had learned in our own minds and gave the group even greater cohesion.

There is within each of us, waiting to be tapped, a wellspring of passion and purpose. What matters isn't which particular activity we engage in, but the effect it has on us. When we follow our bliss, we expand our lives with new meaning. As we become involved in something important to us, our focus and energy flow freely and we often lose ourselves in what we're doing. When we truly desire to do what we are doing, obligation falls away.

Our meaningful activities often entail reaching beyond ourselves, focusing more on our broader connection with others. The volunteer spirit is a good example. People who are excited about their volunteer commitment will talk about its meaning, how their activity helps them see their lives in the context of their communities and the larger world. They are engaged in a broader landscape, and petty hassles and even pain and discomfort diminish because they are absorbed in something meaningful.

Toward the end of my Dad's life, his eyesight faded to the point that he could only read large text in very bright light. Ironically, that is when he volunteered to teach two middle-aged men to read, meeting them twice a week in the library a block from his apartment. Those sessions were highlights in his routine, time spent making new friends and being of help to them. They expanded his life, pulled him out of himself into the broader world. He took great joy from using his own dwindling ability to read, to give a life of reading to two others.

We each contain a strong force that can push us beyond what we ever thought we could do. In some ways we will never be the same after facing chronic illness or significant loss, and perhaps that is exactly what our spirit wants.

The heroes we hear about often emerge from great trials to make their contributions. There are many people, however, who are heroes simply because they live every day with severe physical conditions and work around their limitations to do what they love to do.

Cindi, who has a chronic liver disease, is a good example. One day as we were talking, she shook her head at the fact that her entire life could be filled with doctors' appointments and lab work. But she pours energy into her passion for singing the blues.

When she is with her band on stage belting out a song, she is immersed body and soul in joy as her music engulfs the cheering crowds of her neighbors and friends. It's obvious to everyone that she derives healing energy from following her bliss. On a recent trip to a regional health center where she is on the list for a liver transplant, her doctor told her, "Whatever it is that you are doing, keep it up— it's working wonders."

How do we know the difference between what's meaningful and what drains us or only fills our time? An important signal is that good deep-in-the-gut feeling. When we are in our groove, we are living in the moment. Past and future concerns fade into the background.

Unfortunately for many of us, this is not easy. We have learned through the years that we should place a low priority on doing things just because they feel good. As a consequence, we get mired down in our "to dos" and don't allow our passion to come forward. But it is when our illnesses are challenging that we especially need to follow our bliss, because therein lies a powerful source of energy, healing, and meaning.

As I began to examine why I often get overburdened, I recognized that I have a tendency to respond to opportunities and requests for my time, energy, and talents in a knee-jerk way. I react impulsively, instead of responding thoughtfully. Usually I say "yes" without asking the simple question, "Would I find meaning in this activity?" I realized that if I were to pause, take a deep breath, and ask myself this question,

I would give myself an opportunity to think through my response. I would give an answer that better reflected what is best for me.

We often say "yes" when we really want to decline. We don't want to feel guilty about displeasing someone. We may say, "Sure I'll do it," because we feel that it's our turn. Or we say "of course" when we don't have anything better to do, or to fill what we see as empty space or boredom. All those "yeses" can deplete our time and energy. We may feel flattered to be included, but is it worth the price?

With chronic illness, we don't have unlimited energy to mindlessly react in old ways. But whether we have an illness or not, it's a great gift to ourselves when we say "no" sometimes.

Pursuing meaning in our lives may involve struggle, stress, and pain. It sometimes calls for us to go beyond what we ever thought we could do. It may even result in loss of physical health in exchange for doing something that feeds our spirit.

I had a dear friend named Larry Wagner, who contracted polio in the prime of his life. In some ways he was similar to the actor Christopher Reeve, who was paralyzed by a fall from a horse. Despite the fact that they were both severely limited by their conditions, their lives were illuminated by their passion. Here is Larry's story as told by my husband, Tim.

Before his illness, Larry was a strong and vigorous man. He had two children, ran a successful law practice, and fished and hunted across the Kansas Flint Hills he loved.

Just before the vaccine was available, Larry was stricken with polio, and it almost killed him. It put him permanently into a wheelchair, and required him to use an electric pump to push air through a tube in his mouth so he could breathe and talk. It left him virtually without the ability to move, and it rendered him completely dependent on others to eat, dress, and do just about everything else.

With the help of friends, family, and hired support, Larry moved forward in his life. He maintained his law practice and earned a good living. He transmuted his passions for hunting and fishing into a passion for preserving his own few acres of pristine prairie close to Kansas City, with its ponds and native grasses and buffalo wallow, for the use of naturalists, Boy Scouts, and others to study and enjoy.

Then financial disaster struck. A bank of which he and his father were directors went belly-up, and both Larry and his father lost their investments and life savings.

Although his father was forced into bankruptcy, Larry refused to go that way. He knew that if he embraced the release of bankruptcy, the piece of virgin prairie land he had owned and protected for so long would fall like a ripe plum into the hands of eager developers. The ponds and prairie grasses and buffalo wallows would be replaced with housing developments. So he transferred his property to a foundation, and he fought on.

The federal government and his creditors pushed and demanded and blustered, but he fought on. When his friends who so loved him begged him to release the land, give up the battle that was grinding him down, take out bankruptcy and begin again, Larry still fought on.

It finally got to the point where it seemed as if the battle would kill Larry. The polio that had damaged his body re-asserted itself, and he began failing. His voice became so weak that it was almost impossible to carry on a conversation with him.

Many of his friends who were supporting him by trying to raise the large payments required to stave off the loss of the land, gradually fell away, not out of callousness, but because it was almost unendurably painful to watch him being slowly crushed.

One woman, who had battled alongside Larry throughout, told me that when she had a disturbing dream, she knew she had to get away for awhile or lose her sanity. "I dreamed," she said, "that Larry was drowning in one of the ponds on the place, and I was on the dock trying frantically to assemble his wheelchair, which was in a million pieces. I woke up shivering and crying."

Well, against all odds, Larry won his battle. He convinced the bank that held the note on the land to go far beyond normal banking practices and provide every inch of slack they could. The Nature Conservancy, which had earlier been reluctant to become involved, came up with economic support. And finally the State of Kansas purchased the land, declared it a park, and put in place as board members a few of the passionate protectors who had stuck with Larry through the dark times.

Some of us who had worked with Larry over the years on prairie preservation causes held a reunion one summer at an old Victorian home on the bank of a river in the Kansas Flint Hills. We gathered together that sunny afternoon on the large veranda and I stepped down and snapped a picture, which I later had enlarged and framed.

The magic of that picture flows from the man in the center of the group, the man in the wheelchair. There sits Larry, white hair and whiskers glistening in the sun, so thin that the light almost passes through him, with a look of ecstatic transcendence on his face that is so intense I swear you can see it in the dark.

At first glance the picture is just a snapshot of a group of Kansas folks, gathered together in a pretty spot on a sunny afternoon. If you look closely, however, you'll see in the center a gladiator, a man who won an almost impossible battle. You'll see Larry, shining like the sun.

Larry's passion for his piece of prairie led him to forego comfort and reason. His choice was unique to him. Others, with different passions, will find their place in the world. Each of us needs to look deeply into ourselves to discover our own avenues to joy and fulfillment.

It is all too easy to live our lives just getting by each day. When we open ourselves, though, to finding and following what has meaning, we become at home in the world. And surprisingly, what has meaning is often right in front of us, beckoning with arms wide open.

CHAPTER 8

Bringing Meditative Moments into the Day

"When we lose ourselves in meditative moments, connect with the universe, we open ourselves to healing."

DEBORAH SINGLETON

*M*y body was stiff and sore from the stress and effort of finishing my graduate school finals, and Christmas was only a few days away. I was surrounded by a pile of unwrapped presents and I was overwhelmed. There were still gifts to buy, cooking to do, a tree to decorate, and those were only a few of the urgent tasks on my list.

A familiar wave of martyrdom swept over me as I asked myself why I was always the one who had to do all the holiday preparations. I answered with my usual reply; it was too much trouble to try to get my family to help, and besides it was my job to do these things.

In the past I had always pushed myself through the holiday overload, but the arthritis that had hit me a few months before was making it clear that this year everything would not happen as usual. I just wasn't going to be able to get my body to do the work. Something had to give.

Out of pure necessity I made some changes that Christmas. It wasn't much and it wasn't easy, because my pattern of trying to do it all myself went so deep. I bought fewer gifts and ordered many of them by telephone. Christmas dinner was easier because I reluctantly let others pitch in and help. I cut back on the number of *gatherings I attended, as I saw that being in constant motion, eating foods that weren't good for me, and losing sleep were cumulative drains on my body.*

These changes made me feel guilty and inadequate. They also made me feel out of sync with the world around me. As I watched others race by in their countdown mentalities, I missed being in the familiar flow of their hurried rhythms. I felt like I was missing out on all the fun. But as the holiday progressed I gradually stopped paying attention to that nonsense, and the benefits of slowing down became clear.

I found that in those busy December days, getting rid of planned activities left space for natural pauses. I had time to rest, take a nap, or walk. Because my mind wasn't racing to the usual frenetic drumbeat, I was enjoying people's company more, and recapturing some of the Christmas magic I had almost forgotten.

Over the following years, I have noticed that this slower holiday pace benefits others in my family as well. We all have more time to enjoy the blessings of the season and of each other. One year when my son Matt was home on vacation, the two of us rented several funny movies and just laughed all afternoon, ignoring the ringing telephone and all the seasonal folderol that lurked outside the door.

The benefits have also spread to the rest of the year. When I got over the hump of the difficult but unavoidable decision to slow my holiday, I realized that a slower pace was wonderful. Now, not just during the holidays but throughout the year, I slow down and receive more of what life has to give. In many ways, that Christmas marked the beginning of acceptance of my illness and my understanding of how and why I want to live more in the moment.

Everything has a rhythm. When we are stressed, our bodies speed up with rapid heartbeats and shallow breaths. We slow into an entirely different beat when we are relaxed. The natural world moves to the syncopated rhythm of the seasons. When we moved from the city to a house standing alone in the country, I discovered that I am much more aware of the nature's cycles. I wait each spring for the return of the flashing hummingbirds from a warmer climate, and each fall I watch a nearby lake for ducks gathering to fly south in unison.

Stephan Rechtschaffen, in his book, *Time Shifting,* talks about a process called entrainment, which he believes to be as important as gravity for understanding how our earth works. Entrainment occurs when you place two out-of-sync pendulum clocks side by side, and the next day they'll be keeping time together. It's why salmon travel simultaneously thousands of miles through the sea to the rivers of their birth. For us, it's the process by which we humans fall into synchronization with each other.

Rechtschaffen maintains that entrainment is such an integral part of our lives that we usually don't notice how much it guides our human interactions. We do notice, however, when we or others are out of sync, because it makes us uncomfortable. It's not easy to be quiet, for example, when everyone around us is loud and boisterous. It's why we are annoyed by the slow driver in front of us who pokes along in a fast moving stream of cars.

The concept of entrainment helped me realize how easy it is to become pulled into a frenzied lifestyle without being aware of it. Hyperactivity can become addictive because when our pace is hectic, we can avoid having to face what is actually going on with our lives. Part of the power of the hypnotic rhythm of a frenzied lifestyle is that the fast pace makes us feel important and productive, comfortably in synchronization with the clicking world around us but unaware of the toll it is taking.

As I look back now, I realize that for years before I became ill, part of me yearned for a slower, more contemplative rhythm. I didn't know why I had such a yearning, but now I know I wanted peace and a deeper spiritual existence. Then as my illness emerged, it became clear that I had to slow down and change my ways.

Despite everything zipping around me and my desire to move along at the same pace, my body wasn't cooperating. I was forced to step back and move toward the slower life I had always yearned for at a deeper level. I thought about what I did during my days, and which things I could alter or eliminate to reduce the frenzy.

When I examined my mornings, I realized how I unknowingly set an anxious tone to my day. As I went about my morning preparations, I would listen to news coverage of politics, crime, and the latest disasters. I would often eat breakfast on the move, performing other tasks at the same time. While getting dressed, my mind would be preoccupied with thoughts of what I had to get done. My morning routine was setting me up for tense, over-paced days in which the pain and stiffness of my arthritis would worsen.

I gradually changed my early morning rituals to be quieter and to include meditative moments. The changes weren't necessarily big things—they could be as simple as pauses that connected me to my breath, turning off the news, or reading something uplifting and inspiring.

I still start my days quietly. Perhaps I'll exercise or take a little walk. Whatever the activity, the important thing is to feel more peaceful and in the present. This helps establish a pattern in which I am calmer and more aware of each moment. It gives me the gift of feeling better, moving through my day with less pain.

The way I transition from day to night is just as important. Over the last few years, I've developed a bedtime ritual that relaxes me and allows me to slip more easily into sleep. It is an easy visualization that clears my system of the day's stress.

I get comfortable in bed and close my eyes. I picture myself standing under a gentle waterfall, a beautiful natural place with colorful flowers and green foliage surrounding cascading water.

I take deep breaths as I absorb the sights and sounds around me. I listen to the sound of the gently tumbling water. As the water flows over me, I feel it cleanse and soothe my body from head to toe.

As I stand beneath the flowing stream of water, I slowly scan my body. When I find a tight place, I gently breathe into the tenseness to release it and allow the water to carry it away.

I visualize the water washing away all my cares, until I feel free and transparent. My breath relaxes even more. I am ready to slip gently into sleep.

When we hold the intent to feel more peaceful no matter what our outside circumstances, we find ourselves surrounded by opportunities. Just noticing and observing people who emanate a sense of peacefulness, even strangers, can help us relax into a peaceful moment. I'll never forget one such person we encountered in Hong Kong.

My husband and I were on our way to Bangkok, Thailand, for my son's marriage. We had a few days stopover in Hong Kong, and on our first morning we decided to take a walk in Victoria Park because we had heard it was a place where tai chi was often practiced. We had both been studying tai chi, and wanted to see how the ancient exercise was done in its home country.

Not far from the entrance to the park was a group of six young Chinese women engaged in some sort of movement, but as we neared them we realized that they were doing aerobics to the fast beat of a boom box. That was definitely not what we were looking for.

Some time later we were resting on a bench, when an elderly Chinese gentleman walked by and stopped under a shade tree. He took off his coat and neatly placed it over a nearby fence. For several moments he stood very still with his eyes closed, centering himself.

We were transfixed as he began his tai chi exercise, and his limber body flowed from one graceful and fluid movement to the next. He moved with effortless perfection, each position blended seamlessly into the whole. We later agreed that we could almost see the energy glow around and through him as he slowly shifted and balanced himself through the movements.

When he finished, he stood quietly in place for another minute or two and then put his coat back on and walked away, as if what he had just done were the most common thing in the world. The fatigue from our long trip seemed to vanish. It was a graphic demonstration of how contagious peaceful energy can be.

Another easy and accessible way of feeling more peace is to be in a natural setting and focus on the moment. When our attention is in the now, we are more able to hear a bird sing or see a squirrel run by. Our breathing relaxes and the tension of our body eases. We notice things around us that were invisible while we were stuck in our heads. Tiresome thinking evaporates. In those meditative moments we can feel energy move down through the bottoms of our feet and root us into the earth.

I love to take walks with my friends, but there is a big difference between walking with a friend while you talk about your lives, and walking alone and immersing in the quiet moment. It's possible to share quiet with someone else, but not if either of you can't resist the urge to chatter. The physical exercise might be the same in both instances, but one is distinctly more peaceful.

Nature gives valuable solace and calm in times of turmoil, when we don't know where to go for an emotional anchor. Natural settings allow us to more easily step outside the frenzy of our minds and emotions, and embrace the enduring rhythm of something much larger than ourselves. Entrainment with nature can bring peace into our lives.

My friend Julie's relationship with nature has always been a fundamental part of her life. During a tumultuous time, a neighborhood tree became a symbol for her of finding her own wisdom.

There is a sycamore in the neighborhood park down the hill from my house. It is very old and it leans severely. Even though I grew up in this neighborhood and played in that park my entire childhood, I didn't discover the tree until I was an adult going through a divorce.

With four young children in tow, I moved back to my childhood neighborhood to start anew. To try to get my grounding I began walking one day and there it was, a magnificent sycamore tree that by the laws of physics should have fallen over years ago. But it didn't. It stood strong and full, and how it leaned!

As I struggled with the issues of my divorce, I would visit that tree frequently to remind myself that even though I felt I might fall over, like the tree I had strong roots and was only leaning. Sometimes when I had a critical decision to make I would walk down to my tree, put my hand on its bark and ask the question of the moment. I trusted that the first answer that came to me was the best decision. My tree helped me to start trusting my own intuition.

As I write this years later, I am well past those critical "leaning" moments. But I still live in my old neighborhood and see my tree daily as I drive past, going about the tasks of my life.

I no longer ask important questions while holding on to its bark. I have, for the most part, learned to trust my intuition. Now, I just admire the changing of the seasons with my great leaning sycamore, and sometimes say "thank you" as I pass.

As my illness eases into a less constant companion in my life, I feel a little like Julie. I have fewer critical "leaning" moments. I am freer to trust a life of my own creation, in part because I've learned that at times I need cycles of low energy for my own regeneration.

I know that when I resist a slower rhythm and deny my body the rest and recuperation she needs, I usually create more illness. I have learned to be more patient with myself. I realize the importance of times of lower energy and slower pace to my over-all well-being, even though the "hurry, hurry" mentality occasionally creeps in.

I've learned much about myself in the quiet stillness of meditative moments. Being present in the here and now leads me to a whole new avenue for healing. I feel more of the life of my body and the comfort of my spirit, things that were once distant and alien. I know it is in the stillness of the moment that my true self lives, and it's in stillness that I've learned to love and appreciate the person I found.

CHAPTER 9

Establishing Healing Connections

> We are all angels with only one wing…we
> can only fly embracing each other.
>
> ANONYMOUS

When I first knew I had arthritis, I often complained about how hard it was to turn the key to start my car, open a heavy door, or twist the top off a jar. I grumbled that if people who designed those things had arthritis in their hands, they wouldn't have made them so hard to use.

Luckily I also developed a sharp awareness of others around me who have physical limitations. It was as if I sprouted antennae sensitive to people who go about their lives with fortitude in the face of their daily struggles. Most of those strangers will never know how much they inspired me by their example, and taught me to quit complaining and get on with my life.

One day I found myself behind an elderly man who struggled with a particularly difficult door. After finally getting it open he held it, turned to me with a kind smile, and patiently waited while I went through. It was a small thing but I still remember feeling awash with gratitude, and thinking that if he could smile and be gracious in that situation, I could do the same.

Another stranger who lightened my attitude was a woman about my age who participated with me in a YMCA water exercise class. As our class was gathering for our first session, the rest of us watched her patiently pull herself out of her wheelchair and painstakingly ease herself into the pool. Seeing her move slowly through the water toward our group with a bright smile cheered and helped all of us. I remember her still, and she continues to inspire me.

Recently, when my car was stopped at a traffic light, I noticed a man walking nearby with a cane. He looked as if he were recovering from a stroke and relearning to walk. When he got to the corner curb he stumbled, and it seemed for a moment as if he might tumble forward into the street. Our eyes met briefly as he regained his balance, and we shared a good-natured smile of relief. It was just a brief fleeting contact, but I'm sure we both went on with our spirits a little lighter.

These incidents all share the value of connectedness. It's connection that makes support groups therapeutic and comforting. We usually think of support groups as places where people with similar challenges share stories and solutions. But often their greatest value flows from sharing a smile, seeing a positive outlook, or receiving a kind gesture that says, "I understand and I care. You're not alone."

Chronic illness can foster a sense of isolation. While everyone around us continues life as usual, we are left grappling with major disruptive changes. It's as if we were suddenly attacked by a large animal while everyone else eases down the road unharmed. Why are we the ones the beast picked out?

Our isolation often increases because we don't know how to cope with the accumulating stress that surrounds our illness. We may face strange and uncomfortable tests that could result in disturbing news. A scary symptom might suddenly appear, and doctors and other health personnel may seem remote and uncaring. Connections with friends and family can be disrupted by changes in our routines.

Illness tends to make us more self-focused. It can increase our desire to retreat from the world, as if we need to gather our wagons in a circle for personal safety. If we have a tendency to feel alone, having an illness may cause us to disconnect even more from others.

On the other hand, if we look primarily to others to be our safety net, we will find that no one can truly provide our security. Sometimes we retreat because of the painful gap between the caring and support we hoped to receive from family or friends, and what they are able to give to us.

As always, though, there is a positive side. Our illness can shake us up enough to become more sensitive to healing connections we would formerly have been too busy to notice. This was the case with my friend Kate's sister Gabriel, whose illness opened her to connecting with ten of Kate's friends who lived three thousand miles away. In Kate's words:

When I found out that my sister Gabriel was diagnosed with breast cancer, I wanted to help her in any way I could. As she lives in Vermont and I live in New Mexico, there was the problem of distance. Also, I am a stay-at-home mom with three kids, which made it even more challenging to go help her in Vermont.

I had recently been taught Reiki, a Japanese system that can allow a person to transmit healing energy from a distance to others. In some ways it is much like prayer. An idea came to me to ask my friends to send Reiki to my sister, and to place healing thoughts into small stones that we would send her as well.

I took a small grapevine basket that looked like a bird's nest, placed some special stones from my own collection in it, and passed it around to my friends. When I got the basket back, it was filled with colorful stones and little messages of well-wishes. As I mailed it to my sister, I felt strongly the help and caring the basket contained.

She loved receiving this package and was amazed that there were ten strangers who took time to do something so special for her. Gabriel told me that she kept the nest with the stones near, and would often hold one or rest with them at her side.

When my sister had to go through some very scary tests, she kept telling herself, "I'm getting Reiki, I'm getting Reiki." Just knowing people were sending her healing energy and good thoughts gave her support and comfort to endure it all.

Jill, one of the people who had added her stone to Gabriel's basket, tells about her experience of reaching out to Gabriel:

I took my stone to a mesa top behind my house where at sunrise each morning I practice my yoga and meditation. As I gave myself to the energy of projected healing, there was a crash of thunder, a flash of lightening, and a swift rush of wind heading east toward Kate's sister in Vermont. I felt the land and air giving their support, and felt later when I put my stone into the nest that I was sending the heart of the land with it. I have found that sometimes, when my heart is filled with love and concern for another, the universe responds with charged messages of its own.

This stirring time on the rocks made me think of several lines from one of Gerard Manley Hopkins' poems "God's Grandeur":

*And though the last lights off the black West went
Oh, morning, at the brown brink eastward, springs—
Because the Holy Ghost over the bent
World broods with warm breast and with ah! bright wings.*

Kate said that when Gabriel's husband John was diagnosed with throat cancer two years later, they had someone with a Geiger counter come to their house to check for dangerous radioactive contamination. The man went carefully throughout the house without the instrument ever registering anything. Later, when he was standing by the wood stove talking to Gabriel and her husband, he happened to lift the instrument up beside the shelf with the nest of special stones. To everyone's surprise, the instrument immediately began to click.

They took the basket down from the shelf and tested each stone separately. Not one of the stones individually set off the machine, but when tested collectively the machine again registered a response. The radiation was at such low levels that it was not at all harmful.

The only other thing that set the instrument off, also at a low level, was a large rock out in the yard. A few years earlier a well driller who dowsed the property for water had said that the large rock was very powerful and would be a good place to sit and do meditation. What an amazing thing—the subtle energy of a basket of stones gathered here and there in New Mexico and a meditation rock in Vermont, both having the power to heal and the power to set off a Geiger counter.

Another story of powerful healing connection is described in an upcoming book, *The Bear Is My Father*, written by Bear Heart, a Muskogee Creek medicine man. Bear Heart led an all night Native American Church meeting for his very ill friend, Hector Gomez. A participant in the meeting, Robert Seidenspinner, tells the story.

For Hector, life was hanging in the balance as he was admitted into an intensive care unit in critical condition. He was suffering from internal bleeding due to ruptured blood vessels around his liver.

The night of the meeting, you could feel the energy crackling. Johnny Hernandez took care of the fire and Calvin Magpie's son took care of the drum. Bear Heart took charge of the meeting in a very focused way.

From early on he let us know that this was a healing meeting and we were praying for a man's life. Bear Heart told us that he wanted us to see Hector not as he was at the moment, in the hospital on various levels of life support, but as we knew him in other ways; smiling, laughing, happy, and enjoying himself. Bear Heart directed each of us to call upon a vision of Hector as healthy, strong, and full of life. As Bear Heart set this tone, something deep inside me knew we were on the correct path and this was definitely going to be a healing ceremony.

That night we prayed all night long, sang, and ate medicine. The meeting was powerful, and soon after, Hector took a turn for the better. He had a procedure done and came out of the coma.

Another big miracle was that he was put on the list of those to receive a liver transplant, despite the fact that he had no money or medical insurance. In fact, at the time he was placed on the list, he was not even an official citizen of the United States. Hector Gomez had prayer in his life and it worked for him.

Some of our most healing connections are those that lighten us up. There's nothing quite like a spontaneous laugh to help us let go of cares, but it's hard to experience laughter when we're alone. When we're with light-hearted friends, the healing power of laughter can work wonders.

When I asked Linda what helps her live easier with chronic pain, she told me the story of discovering the magical power of laughter to diminish her discomfort and lift her spirit:

When I was younger and would rank the priorities in my life, fun was often near the bottom of the list. But in the past ten years, I have learned to put it way, way closer to the top. There is great truth in the expression "laughter is the best medicine."

I will never forget a flare-up that caused a lot of swelling and pain in my knees. Walking was difficult so I was inclined to cancel a trip to Las Vegas that had been planned with several friends. My husband supported my decision either way and said if I wanted to go, we could just lie low when we got there. It was a five-hour drive, and the five of us decided to take turns telling jokes along the way. I don't think I have ever laughed so much in my life!

Anyway, here's the miracle. By the time we arrived, the pain and inflammation were so much less that I was able to walk up and down the strip for the entire weekend. That was the time I learned about the power of endorphins—the more you laugh and have fun, the more they go out to your body like little messengers of instant healing.

Some of the most fascinating studies on healing connections explore the health benefits we gain from our pets. Many of us know from our own experiences with a cat or dog that they can counteract loneliness and lighten our hearts with unconditional love, but we now know that our pets actually change our body chemistry.

An article titled "Tails of Love," by Geoff Brown, which appeared in the November/December 2009 issue of *AARP Magazine*, put it this way:

"When a person interacts with a pet, the central nervous system releases several hormones that cause feelings of pleasure—and one hormone in particular, oxytocin, appears to play a major role in reinforcing the bond. Produced by new mammalian mothers to encourage bonding with their offspring, oxytocin creates a sense of warmth, nurturing, and calm. In 2002 two South African researchers measured oxytocin levels not only in humans petting dogs but in the dogs themselves: the dogs experienced the same chemical releases and calming effects as did the humans."

Our pets give us opportunities to express our love through the daily care and affection they need. It's almost impossible not to be brightened by their playfulness and companionship.

I experienced this bond with our old dog Walter, a Basset/Labrador mix. A primary task in Walter's life was to remind me each day to go for a walk with him.

One summer afternoon we were walking along a dirt road near our house, and Walter in his usual exploratory mode trotted out ahead of me, around a bend and out of sight. When I got past the bend, I almost stumbled on a rattlesnake moving off the road toward the bushes. In a panic I called for Walter, and when I finally found him, his mouth was foaming from being bitten by the snake a few moments earlier. My husband and I rushed him to the vet and Walter put up a valiant effort. But his aging body couldn't overcome the snake's venom, and he died several days later.

On a visit a few weeks after Walter's death, our friend Bear Heart held a small ceremony for him around a fire one evening. After he had chanted and placed sage and other things in the fire, he told me that Walter had protected me from the snake by putting himself in harm's way; he had chosen to be bitten in my place.

Whether Walter saved me from the rattlesnake bite or not, he was and is a healing presence in my life. I often look out my window and see the rock marking the place where his ashes lie. I know his spirit is still around.

Our pets are uniquely suited to pull us outside of ourselves. They give us physical intimacy, constant affection, and undemanding companionship. They love us without judgment, which allows us to relax into exactly who we are. Without them the world would be a much less open-hearted and happy place.

Every day we are surrounded with opportunities to lift our spirits. We may find them where we expect them to be, but they also lie in wait in surprising and unusual places. When we hold ourselves open to their power to heal, it's as if there is a "new normal" operating in our lives.

Our lives can be enhanced by being open to strangers living their courage, prayer aligning us with healing energies, laughter lightening our load, pets giving us love, and all the other myriad forces surrounding us with chances to grow and heal. We each have great power to increase our health, reduce our discomfort, and boost our attitude by increasing our healing connections. Here are a few questions to ask yourself as you think about the healing connections in your life:

❖ Do I often enjoy a good laugh or make someone else laugh or smile?

❖ Do I often reach out to touch others in need?

❖ Do I take heart from those around me who show courage?

❖ Am I around people who are generally positive and upbeat and see the best in me? Do I see the best in them?

If you answered "no" to some of these questions, you might want to create opportunities that will allow you to change your answers. Identify some healing connections—people, activities, animals, plants, places—that will strengthen and enrich your life, and then make those connections. We do fly when we embrace each other.

CHAPTER 10

Discovering Mystery and Possibility

"'There's no use trying,' Alice said. 'One can't believe impossible things.' 'I daresay you haven't had much practice,' said the Queen. 'When I was your age, I always did it for half-an-hour a day. Why, sometimes I've believed as many as six impossible things before breakfast.'"

LEWIS CARROLL,

THROUGH THE LOOKING GLASS

Braced against the cold Peruvian rain, we stood with a tour group comprised of people from all over the world. My husband Tim, our friend Deborah, and I were barely able to hear our guide talk over the noise of the rain pounding on the thatched roof above us. Here we stood in the middle of Machu Picchu, an enormous city built by the Incans in the fifteenth century and once the most important spiritual center of the Inca Empire. Now we could only use our imaginations because the rain and cloud cover hid its majestic mountain peaks, green terraces, and ancient metropolis of perfectly fitted stones.

While we had climbed slippery stone steps to reach the hut where we now stood, I wondered whether my knees could make it through this arduous day. If any one of us had suggested stopping, the others would probably have jumped at the chance, even though we had come many miles to be here and were each reluctant to call it quits.

While our guide talked to us about views we couldn't see, I asked myself, "Can I really do this?" Visions of injuring myself and being airlifted out of this remote place filled my mind, but I somehow trusted my reassuring voice. I was willing to take my own advice either way. My quiet response was, "Don't think about all you're going to do. Take one step at a time and focus only on that step."

As the day went on, the rain gradually stopped, and we began to experience the mystical somber beauty that the gray overcast skies lent to this amazing place. At one juncture our guide gave us the choice to climb rock stairs to a lookout point, or to take a lower route. Those of us who took the lower path soon found ourselves in an emerald green meadow sprinkled with blue forget-me-nots and a pair of munching, unconcerned llamas. In the magic of that moment I felt a wave of appreciation for my body, for weathering the obstacles and allowing me to experience this day.

It's hard to know when I first noticed that the familiar pain and heavy stiffness in my knees were gone, but it had happened some time during the morning. Although several parts of my body had been affected by arthritis, my knees had been the hardest hit. It is where my symptoms first surfaced, and over the years they had consistently caused problems and restrictions. But here I was in the jungles of Peru with knees that felt healthy and strong.

At the same time that my knees had lightened, Deborah was feeling her knees get heavier and stiffer, as if some rapid aging process had taken over. She is a spiritual teacher who does healing work, and she had temporarily taken into her knees the painful energy from mine. Some healers pull the sickness or pain out of a person they are working on and hold it temporarily in their bodies. This is what she did for me.

The limitations and pain slowly returned a day or so later, but not as severely. In Machu Picchu, I had been startled out of the painful body pattern in my knees by a healing surprise of normal movement. I realize now that I must have been open enough for this to happen. In that miraculous time, I experienced what it felt like to have normal knees. Deborah gave me a glimpse into a new vision for my health.

After returning from Peru, I thought a great deal about how I had forgotten the feel of healthy knees. My experience in Peru gave me a glimmer of hope that perhaps I had other options than a life sentence of rheumatoid arthritis. Up to that point, I had unconsciously agreed with the medical establishment that over time my health would decline, or at best stay the same. It never occurred to me that there was any other possibility. Doesn't the term "chronic illness" imply forever?

The experience helped me realize, in a very concrete way, that there is an essence in disease behind its physical presence, just like there is an essence in each of us behind our physical presence, and that if the essence of the disease is removed, the disease cannot remain. I still haven't worked it all out but I know, somehow, that this is one place where hope resides.

I talked to Deborah later about what had happened in Machu Picchu and she described her work as holding a vision for others, so that their own healing capabilities can be enhanced. She sees herself in a partnership to support the body's innate intelligence. This extraordinary experience gave me an appreciation of the importance of having people around us who carry for us a healing vision.

I always had strong trust and hope in most aspects of my life, but when it came to my health I automatically expected the worst. I had lived with the belief that I would have a lifetime of illness since the day I was diagnosed with arthritis.

I would regularly go through times of floating anxiety, when I worried about what was going to happen next. The anxiety would usually settle on whatever part of my body was bothering me the most. One morning, for instance, it might be focused on my hands.

Should I get a splint? Was it time to ask my doctor about different medications or treatments? Did my fingers need another operation? Why was this happening to me? What did I do wrong?

Anxious thoughts dominated me and cancelled out any consideration of trying simple things that might help my hands feel better, such as gently rubbing them, using hot or cold packs, or resting them because I may have worked them too hard.

Although my experience in Peru with my knees had given me a new vision of my health, the familiar old anxieties and feelings of hopelessness continued. Because my mother and stepmother had slow painful deaths, at some level I believed that I would suffer the same fate.

But now there was something different. I *had* experienced the lifting of pain in my knees, even after I had strenuously climbed a mountain of steps. I had, at least briefly, taken a significant turn toward new possibilities.

There is enormous power in what we believe. Our beliefs orchestrate our lives. Our daily activities, the people we gather around us, and the lives we create are to a great extent determined by our beliefs.

Expansive beliefs that allow us to be open to change and receptive to good things draw positive people and experiences toward us. Just as importantly, openness allows us to recognize and embrace opportunities when they do come along.

If, on the other hand, our beliefs focus on a world that is contracted and closed, they attract and hold negativity. Because of thought patterns and beliefs, we may resist opportunities and pull darkness toward us. Because they don't fit with our beliefs about the nature of the world, we may even reject obvious blessings staring us right in the face.

There is a story of a devout man who found himself stranded in a flood on the roof of his house. Because of his religious devotion, he was certain that God would rescue him.

After awhile his neighbor came along in a boat and offered to take him to safety, but he said, "No, I don't need your help. I know God will save me." The water rose higher but he believed that God wouldn't let him drown, so when a helicopter came to lift him to safety, he refused. "No! I'm waiting to be saved by God," he yelled, and the helicopter went away.

Eventually the water rose above his head, and he drowned and found himself in the presence of God. "I had faith in you," he said. "Why didn't you save me?" "What are you talking about?" God replied. "I sent you a boat and a helicopter."

Richard Wiseman, a British professor of psychology at the University of Hertfordshire, studied why some people seem to have all the luck in life, while others are "magnets for ill fortune." His research affirms that so-called lucky people perceive more options and are more open to the positive world around them.

Wiseman's studies confirm that most luck is not random. He estimates that only 10% of luck is chance, while 90% is "actually defined by the way we think."

A person, for instance, who has to wait for a long time in a doctor's office may find in a magazine article a solution to a problem he is facing, while another person in the same waiting room sits stone-faced and stewing because the doctor is keeping him waiting. Is the first person luckier than the second? To a large extent, luck is often no more than being willing to take life in stride and take advantage of the possibilities that arise.

Change, such as altering thought patterns, can be unsettling because it involves risk. I think back to a friend who, whenever I offered him a new perspective on a situation that was bothering him, would always respond with an immediate "Yes, but it won't work because...."

I'm sure some of my suggestions were better than others, but his automatic negative reaction didn't allow him to consider them at all.

His blanket resistance closed the door, denying him room for new options, ideas, and insights.

Observing my friend's reaction to new ideas helped me learn to listen for my own "Yes, buts," whether I say them aloud or think them to myself. I examine my own reaction to see whether my "Yes, but" is a preface to considering the desirability of a new idea, or just resistance to change.

Some people maintain their hopeful, receptive attitudes through the most difficult of times. Even in the direst circumstances, the peace that hope produces can go a long way toward allowing us to live each day to its fullest. Two friends of mine, Carol and Lisa, told me how hope supports them.

Carol is an artist who has multiple sclerosis. As we talked about how she lives with her illness, she said:

> *I don't think about where my MS will take me five years from now, I think about what I'm going to do today. Some days I wake up and I can't do very much, but on many days I have the energy to paint. I can no longer paint fine detail because I don't have the steady hand I used to rely on for my exacting work. But now my art is freer—my hand makes freer strokes. My paintings are less perfectly made, but more from my heart.*

When I visited Lisa, my neighbor who has lung cancer, I was expecting to see someone beaten down by her situation. I knew she had suffered through a series of chemotherapy sessions over the last six weeks, and after one of the sessions had almost died.

But there sat Lisa in her bright living room, with the sun lighting her smiling face. She mentioned an upcoming chemotherapy session, but for most of the visit she talked about her new project of learning Hebrew. "It's slow going," she said, "but I have always wanted to learn this language, and maybe even go someday to Israel. There's no better time than the present."

Carol and Lisa are wonderful teachers for me of the value of hope, no matter what our circumstances. I know that with hope I can create my own healing space in the here and now. None of us knows what any of our futures will bring, but we do know that when we stay open and receptive, healing surprises can happen.

Try this exercise to help you open to new possibilities:

———⊶⊷———

Go to a quiet, comfortable place. Close your eyes and relax into your breathing. Feel your body and mind at ease and receptive.

Think about a troubling situation in your life. Allow thoughts and feelings to come to the surface. Are they all worried, anxious, negative? Are there some among them that are hopeful, open to new opportunities?

If there are positive thoughts, bring them to the front of your mind. Imagine other hopeful aspects of the situation and bring those into your mind as well.

Remind yourself that a troubling situation often can have a positive outcome because of possibilities that you never thought of or anticipated.

Focus on your breath and hold the troubling situation gently in your mind, surrounded by hope and awareness of possible positive outcomes.

Release the situation from your mind, breathe easily, and open your eyes.

Each day, practice believing impossible things.

CHAPTER 11

Seeing the Gifts

"If the only prayer you say in your whole life
is 'thank you,' that would suffice."

MEISTER ECKHART

*W*hile *visiting friends Tony and Dorothy
in Los Alamos, we had a little outing one afternoon to meet Tony's
mother. We had heard many tales about her life and the good things
she had done for others and her community over the years, and we
wanted to meet her. Our friends drove us through a shady neighbor-
hood of small, well-kept homes to her house. We walked up the ramp
to her front door, knocked, and went in.*

*She greeted us with a welcoming smile from where she sat in
her wheelchair in her living room. Although her son had told us
that she had significant discomfort and pain, it didn't show. Ninety-
seven years old and barely ninety pounds, she was bone on bone.
She looked as if she had been stripped to her essence, and it was in
her essence that she lived.*

*Her bright greeting drew us into a room filled with pictures and
treasures from her life and travels—carved Thai dancers, Southwest
oil paintings by her son Tony, and a hand-crafted blanket chest that
her husband, long passed away, had built when he was fourteen.*

*We talked of many things that summer afternoon. She told us
about her trips, especially to South Africa which was her favorite
destination. We admired her tiny garden just outside her patio door,
colored with marigolds, petunias, and roses. Her face brightened as*

she described her current project of writing her memoirs; how much pleasure she was discovering in revisiting events and people who had filled the many years of her life. She mentioned with a small sigh that the day before, her hands had gotten so weak that she had had to stop long before she had planned, but she was going to get back to her typewriter that very afternoon.

She sparkled as she talked about how grateful she was to have her son and daughter-in-law living a few blocks away, and to have a woman who came each day to take care of her needs so she could stay in her home.

I could see that her gratefulness was a natural part of who she was. It fed her with energy and a reason to be alive. Her life was far from easy. Her daughter was estranged, she was widowed, and she had suffered from pain for the last few years. I knew it took a great deal of strength for her to visit with us. But I also knew that in sharing herself, she found joy.

Later I saw a picture taken on that day, all of us surrounding her in her wheelchair. What surprised me was how small and frail she looked in the photograph; not at all how I remembered her when I was in her presence. Our camera didn't capture the expansiveness of her grateful heart.

Everyone experiences times of difficulty, but a strong current of gratitude creates special and resilient people who search out the gifts in their lives, no matter how painful their situation may be. Of course we all sometimes get mired down by life and become sour toward the world, but it's important to not remain there. If we stay in the darkness too long we become filled with it until we overflow with bitterness, which then spreads like an emotional plague to others.

It may not seem like it at the time, but even in our darkest hours we can search our world and find reasons to feel grateful. Some people do this more naturally than others, but with commitment it is something that we each can learn to do to lift our lives. In the depths of pain and loss, we can be filled with gratitude.

At this writing, Julie, a friend of mine, is taking care of her elderly mother and feeling the stress of emotional and physical demands. At the same time that her mother's needs are increasing, she has to deal with her own chronic condition, which is especially affected by stress. She told me that in the midst of it all, she draws strength from her gratitude for her relationship with her mother and how much she herself is growing. Here in her own words is Julie's story:

I am currently in the process of making decisions concerning my ninety-two-year-old mother, who seems to be fading away as she grows frailer and more forgetful. It is sad to watch and I am grieving for this painful loss, but at the same time there is much for which to be thankful—the close relationship we have enjoyed, the wisdom she has imparted to me, the example of steadfast courage she has lived, and her spunky independence—the list is long and her legacy is rich.

As my mother and I move into the awkward and confusing role reversal of child and parent, I am thankful for others who have been here before me, offering helpful suggestions and comfort and empathy—a dear friend who is a social worker, another who works in the field of gerontology, and a neighbor who is experiencing the same thing with her mother.

Most of all I am grateful for what I am discovering about my mother and myself. I am gaining a gentler approach toward my mother and others. I am in a bittersweet time, and I savor the experiences it contains with gratitude.

As Julie works through her shifting relationship with her mother, she is discovering that she has to deal with her situation at various levels. On one level she has to manage her own health issues, at the same time that her mother's needs are becoming more complicated and stressful. She needs to maintain her own physical and emotional balance so she doesn't deplete her energy.

On another level, Julie wants to do "the right things" as she makes decisions concerning her mother. This is especially challenging because their relationship has turned upside down. She has become more parent than child, yet to the extent possible she wants to respect her mother's wishes for independence.

During this difficult and complex time, Julie doesn't fill with anger and resentment. Although those emotions probably do rise to the the surface at moments, they are not dominant notes in her emotional mix. Gratitude is the dominant note. It allows her deeper appreciation and respect for her mother, and for her own steps toward becoming a gentler and more patient person.

It may seem illogical to work on our personal growth while we are in the midst of hard times, but as with Julie, it is challenging times that require us to dig deeper within ourselves to find new sources of strength and trust. When life is going smoothly, there is less motivation to look inward. Difficulties force us to grow and evolve by putting us in territory where there are no easy answers.

A key step toward experiencing more gratitude is to address the negative experiences, and the judgments and resentments they create, that we all carry inside. They are often hidden away with other negatives in our secret life: unkind things we did toward others; situations where we failed; and generalized feelings of anger, resentment, and self-doubt.

Just as it's important to release emotions that block movement toward growth and peace, it's also important to release them in order to experience gratitude. We can't feel grateful for the blessings in our life when we are immersed in resentment, yearning, and fear.

If we are filled with anger at the way life has mistreated us, we can't appreciate the beauty of the light sparkling on the dewy grasses outside our window. If our stomachs are tight with anxiety about our illness, we can't feel a glow of happiness for the love of our family. While we are aching with desire for strength or wealth or success, we aren't able to experience the quiet satisfaction of an open-hearted moment with a friend.

There is a Buddhist story about a man who was searching for spiritual wisdom. He walked many miles to meet with a wise teacher and hear his words, so he could feel the peace and happiness he desperately wanted. Instead of speaking, though, the teacher offered him a cup of tea. To the man's dismay, as the teacher poured the tea he didn't stop when the cup was full but kept pouring until it flowed over the brim and onto the table.

When the man asked the wise teacher why he did this, the teacher responded that the visitor's cup was already so full of negativity, that there was no room for anything new and fresh. The man needed to come back when his cup was empty.

Hard times are like that teacher—they have a way of forcing us to examine our cup of beliefs and experiences, so we can get rid of some of them to make room for new attitudes and tools. Reducing the negativity in our cup and replacing it with gratitude should be high on our list, but it's not easy because those dark pieces of us are strong. They are deeply imbedded in our perception of the world. This is particularly true during difficult times, when positivity can feel false and foreign. With commitment and practice, however, a fundamental shift can happen. When we act "as if," over time, gratitude can become our truth.

A good place to begin is to focus on appreciation for our journey of discovery and assure ourselves that whatever we need will be there for us at the right time. When we can hold our hearts open and trusting and curious, new insights as well as people come to help us along the way.

The path to gratitude is one of those "bad news/good news" things. Although it can be very difficult to rid ourselves of negative emotions, sometimes just feeling gratitude is strong enough to push them out, at least for a short time. In those brief moments of respite from yearning or fear, we can experience how good it is to feel grateful.

We've all had moments when a stunning sunset has blown our minds clear of negative chatter, for instance, or a touch or kind word from a loved one has stilled our fear. Along with the joy in beauty or the comfort of love, there always runs gratefulness.

The current of gratitude we build into our lives will be stronger and more resilient if it is accompanied by a deepening connection to our inner world, and that's something we can do in many ways. Some of the things I do to connect are pay attention to my dreams and what they tell me, quiet myself away from the noisy world, and imagine creating the changes I desire. We can draw, play music, or write poetry. We can work with a therapist or garden or meditate. We can saunter through the woods, talk to a friend, or explore our feelings in a journal.

There are teachers who can provide insight, fellow travelers to share our journey and reflect our inner strengths and beauty, and books filled with the experiences and lessons of others. However we do it, as we become more attuned to our deeper self, we become more aware of our fundamental values. It is those values that are the platform on which our gratitude rests.

The power of old hurts and yearnings for externalities will fade as the strength of what's important to our heart emerges. We'll be more sensitive to how we feel when we are around certain people or doing certain things. We will listen intuitively and know if what we are doing and people we are with support our healing.

If we have the commitment to heal our wounds and honor our feelings, healing will happen. As re-alignment with our inner selves occurs, more and more of our moments become infused with gratitude.

A few years ago during a particularly discouraging time in my life, I had a dream that shifted my whole attitude. Like many people

I ignored my dreams because they didn't seem significant, but early one morning this dream literally woke me up with my heart pounding, and I've never forgotten it.

The dream was simple. I saw before me two high sandstone mesas with a deep canyon cutting between them. On the top of each mesa was a large hand. The hands were facing each other and throwing an infant back and forth across the canyon, as if they were playing catch with a ball. With each toss, the baby barely made it across. Finally, on one throw the baby didn't reach the hand on the other side, and I watched in horror as it plummeted toward the canyon floor. Amazingly, the moment before the baby hit the ground, two gigantic hands rose from the bottom of the canyon and caught the infant, safe and secure.

As I thought about the dream, I realized that although it left me breathless, it was also reassuring. The one thing I remembered reading about dreams was that everyone in them represents an aspect of the dreamer, and that felt especially true as I thought about my baby dream.

I realized that the baby symbolized how I often felt about myself; vulnerable yet full of life. Both sets of hands, though, were also parts of me, and it was a little harder to understand what they represented. Eventually, like a picture snapping into focus, the significance of the hands suddenly became clear.

The tossing hands were my desire to move forward and try new things, even though there may be risk. The hands at the bottom were my strong, deeper self and values, there to cushion my falls.

The dream was telling me that I didn't need to worry so much about the risk of new things, because the strength in my center would protect me. It was saying that even though circumstances can be unpredictable and dangerous, I contain a safety net woven into my core.

To this day when I remember the dream, I feel gratitude. In one fell swoop it took away much of the fear I carried around, and allowed room in my cup for more peace and thankfulness.

Gratitude grows naturally when we abandon old negative feelings and beliefs, and become more in touch with our essential truths. As we clear the way for a higher dimension to all of our experiences, each day becomes more permeated with gratefulness.

A friend wrote about how he intentionally creates more gratitude in his days:

A few years ago an Indian friend told me that every morning he would face the rising sun, and with a prayer in his own language, thank the sun for the coming day. Since then I often do something similar. I turn toward the sun and say, "Thank you for this day," and it subtly but powerfully improves what follows. When I remember to do my little ceremony, my days tend to be happier and easier. They contain less anxiety, and go onto the plus side of my ledger.

I think the reason this works for me is that it starts off my day tuned to a place of gratitude. By blessing my day before it happens, I position myself to see the gifts and messages of things, even things that are painful, difficult, or disappointing. When I declare without reservation that the day is good before it occurs, good is what usually happens.

Many cultures contain traditions and daily practices of gratefulness. While traveling on the island of Bali in Indonesia, I noticed that many taxis had small baskets on their dashboards containing a fresh flower, some grains of rice, and a few blades of cut grass. Then I began to notice those baskets everywhere: in front of stores and residences, in hotel lobbies, and on roadsides. These were offerings that were performed first thing in the morning, as a way to bless the new day.

Whether spiritual practices of gratitude are a morning prayer, a basket of offerings, or a morning kiss, they all open us to the awareness that our lives contain bright gifts. We don't know exactly what each new day will bring, but when we approach it with openness and appreciation, we are ready to be pleasantly surprised because we are less likely to be burdened by negatives.

This soul searching and inner work can be challenging and uncomfortable. It may seem like more than we can do, when it's all we can do to just get through the day. Over time though, as our process unfolds, our self-exploration shines a loving light on what once diminished us. Our eyes open to the gifts and teachings that are inherent in our difficult experiences. Our days get easier and begin to blossom with gratitude.

Appreciation feels good because it opens our hearts. Try this appreciation exercise:

Find a quiet place where you are alone.
Close your eyes and follow your breath as it flows easily in and out.
Place your hand over your heart and feel its steady beat.
Expand your heart to include a circle of caring people in your life.
Imagine one special person from the circle coming forward, and feel your hearts connect.
Appreciate all that person is to you.
Breathe in the grateful feelings and the loving connection.
Rest awhile in the glow of gratitude.
The next time you are with that person, give voice to your feelings.

CHAPTER 12

Coming Home

"Just keep coming home to yourself. You are
the one you have been waiting for."

BYRON KATIE, *LOVING WHAT IS*

*M*y eyes opened to the dawn light filter-
ing through the hotel windows in Winslow, Arizona. Today was my
birthday, and as my husband slept quietly beside me, my drowsy
mind wandered through memorable birthdays of the past. I have
always felt there was a special power to birthdays; they seem to have
childlike hope woven into them. That day the world is wide open.

As I lay in the early morning time, I pondered what I wanted
for the coming year. Even though asking myself that question on my
birthday was a tradition for me, it felt particularly important right
then. What did I really want?

The first thing that came to mind was to rid myself of the burdens
of rheumatoid arthritis. I was feeling my usual early morning pain,
but today it was combined with the bone-deep weariness of dealing
every day with this painful disease. But as I focused on making a
birthday wish for something new, my discouraging thoughts faded
and my spirits lifted.

I thought about all the progress I had made. I wondered if some-
how my magical wish were to come true and I were given back the
health of earlier times, would I automatically fall into my old pat-
terns? Would I tuck away most of what I had learned and slip again
into being overly involved in the lives of other people? Would I find

myself mindlessly running again through my days like a chicken with her head cut off? Would I lose the connection with my body for which I had worked so hard? Most importantly, would my deepened spiritual life fade away?

As I floated in the midst of those questions, I felt a strong sense that the answer to all of them was "no." I would keep growing. I wouldn't even be tempted to revert to my old ways.

At the same time I was affirming my appreciation for my growth through the years with arthritis, I wondered why I still felt upset and agitated. I yearned for a stronger center, one that generated more peace and guidance to help deal with my outside world.

I gradually realized that part of my problem was that I had let my physical limitations seep into other areas of my life. I had developed a subconscious belief that because I was physically limited, I was limited in other aspects of my being. No matter what was happening, I would not have enough energy to be who I wanted to be.

I had acquired an automatic response of "I can't," which meant that I usually couldn't. It wasn't that I cared so much about keeping up with everyone around me—it was more that I had let my physical restrictions contaminate my self-image, so I felt lessened as a person.

I thought about how the limitations I had gradually placed on myself were accumulating. Something Parker Palmer said in his book, Let Your Life Speak, *came to my mind: "No punishment anyone might inflict on us could possibly be worse than the punishment we inflict on ourselves by conspiring in our own diminishment."*

It was clear to me that if I truly wanted to live more completely from the peace and assurance of my center, I needed to release an accumulation of judgments about myself. I had to unravel years of letting my illness define who I was.

This birthday morning contained a very special gift. I had awakened with a deeply felt wish. I wanted to have more peace and self-assurance; I wanted to define myself by my strengths, not my weaknesses. Just feeling that desire gave me an inkling of the power I had to alter how I inhabited my life.

My realization that morning was somewhat ironic. To a great extent, the growth and deepening spiritual connection I had developed at that point had happened because I had shifted my personal definition away from people and events outside of me and had moved more to my center. I had learned that if I wanted to have more peace and strength, I had to find them within myself.

I had not, however, paid enough attention to how my own attitudes were contaminating me from inside. I went back over the process in my mind that had helped me overcome defining myself through the judgments and criticisms of others.

Chronic illness causes most of us to rely more heavily on other people. When we're weakened and frightened, we tend to turn outward for support. There is nothing wrong with that, as long as we don't give up our own authority to decide who and what we are.

Our relationships with others come and go and shift over time. Our relationship with ourselves is forever. Our inner being is always there to provide us with support and encouragement. Marcus Aurelius centuries ago spoke this truth: "When jarred unavoidably by circumstances, revert at once to yourself, and don't lose the rhythm more than you can help. You'll have a better grasp of the harmony if you keep on going back to it."

Sometimes, becoming uncomfortable and "jarred" enough, as I did on that birthday morning, is what it takes to send us inside to the constancy in our centers. When we are in our center, in that position of safety and love, we can find uncritical understanding of who we are, and decide for ourselves how we would like to be.

Don Miguel Ruiz writes in *The Voice of Knowledge,* that each of us has a story that we create over the course of our lives. He sees our parents and others as storytellers who taught us early lessons about what to believe about ourselves, so that their stories about us became the basis for our own stories. As adults, Ruiz says, we need to unlearn some of our early lessons because they diminish us as a person. When we shed others' stories about us, we have space to create a new narrative that defines us by our inner strength rather than by others' opinions.

It could be, for instance, that our parents repeatedly corrected us by emphasizing our limitations and faults or by comparing us to others who did better. Or perhaps we grew up with persistent criticism and teasing from siblings and schoolmates. These early influences can become central to how we see ourselves when we are grown.

Often in families where criticism predominates, there is an underlying tendency to avoid being criticized ourselves by blaming others when things go wrong. When that happens, we may absorb a double whammy. Combined with low self-esteem from a childhood of criticism, we may be inclined to give other people responsibility over our lives by blaming them for our difficulties. This makes it very hard to find the power to positively redefine who we are.

On the other hand, most of us also had family members, friends, teachers, or neighbors who emphasized the good things they saw in us. They helped us build on our strengths and highlighted our qualities and talents. They encouraged us to internalize a story in which we saw and relied on our strengths.

Thanks to their influence, when we are confronted with challenges and problems, we are more likely to see ourselves able to cope, because they instilled in us a story in which we are good and competent people.

I recently attended a memorial service for a man named Rocco at which we celebrated the contributions he brought to our small community. Almost until the day he died, he put together and directed plays and musical productions for all ages at our local arts center.

His memorial service was filled with stories by friends and neighbors about how much Rocco had given to the community, especially to young people whose talents and self-confidence had blossomed under his care. One girl spoke movingly about how he had encouraged her performances in the plays he directed. She remembered that he would say, "Don't worry about forgetting your lines, just hold in your heart what the play is saying. Even if you have to invent a few lines, it will be fine."

She talked about how thankful she was that Rocco saw what she was capable of doing long before she saw it in herself. Even though she didn't think of it in those terms, she was grateful that Rocco had helped her write her story so it contained healthy dollops of competence and creativity.

Our stories belong to us, and they grow throughout our lives. We add chapters and other pieces to them as our lives unroll, but we can also go back and change what is already there. A big part of our power over our lives comes from understanding that we have stories about who we are, figuring out just what they contain, and deciding if we want them to be different. We are the narrators. We can control our own stories.

A dear friend once talked to me about her intent to go to a new therapist because her old therapist didn't see her as strong and capable. "I don't think I can tell the same old story about what the doctors did to me one more time," she said. "It makes me tired even thinking about it!" She has realized that she has a story, and she is ready to begin editing it so that it better serves her needs.

Some changes are more difficult than others, of course. It's usually fairly easy to alter the way we interpret facts and events because they are external to us. It is harder to change our perception of ourselves as participants in those events.

I once attended a workshop where I learned at a very personal level to appreciate how adversity develops our strengths and abilities. One of the exercises during the workshop was to compile a list of challenges and setbacks that we had faced in the past or were currently experiencing, and then share our list with others in the class. The stories ran the gamut—illness, divorce, death of loved ones, loss of jobs, bouts of depression, and abuse. The heaviness in the room was palpable as person after person shared their deep hurts and disappointments.

Next, we broke up into pairs and described to each other our tales of living through our difficulties. We took turns telling our own story, then listening to our partner's story and finding the inner qualities that shined through the struggles.

After I described my story of arthritis and divorce, my partner spontaneously said: "You're living a life of courage!" I can still feel today how her words touched and encouraged me.

Before that moment, I would have described myself as someone who had just muddled through those tough times. With that simple remark, my partner helped me see myself in a fundamentally different way. She showed me how to understand my story from a more loving perspective.

Since then, when I need extra encouragement to face a new obstacle, I repeat her exact words to myself. Doing this reminds me of my strength and helps me face the challenges that come.

When it was my partner's turn, she described her anguish as she went through a series of job losses, financial problems, and a divorce. When I asked her about what was happening in the present, she described a new job she really liked, a hiking club that she enjoyed, and the stimulating new people she was meeting.

It was clear that she was moving from a series of painful chapters into ones full of promise. We talked about how her difficulties had given her a deep resilience that allowed her to enter her next stage with vitality and self-confidence.

We both ended the exercise with a new understanding of our strengths and a realization that the hardships we had faced had, in retrospect, also been opportunities. We gained a greater appreciation of ourselves as people who during hard times had grown in courage and resilience.

When the group reconvened, everyone discussed how meaningful it had been to share our histories. We had been used to telling our stories simply as struggles. We learned that we had been leaving out the most important parts: how we had grown through struggle. We placed new frames around old pictures of our past, giving our stories new meaning.

Although we often deny it, we have great power over our lives. But in order to exercise that power in ways that enhance us, we have to know who we are and see our own goodness. Psychologist Carl Rogers reminds us that: "The curious paradox is when I accept myself just as I am, then I can change."

A wonderful way to increase our understanding of ourselves is to think of everyone around us as mirrors. It is amazing how what we experience on the inside is reflected in the world around us.

Our surroundings change day to day and moment by moment, in sync with our own thinking and feelings. If we wake up for instance with a dark cloud hanging over us, we may notice that many of the people we encounter through the day are grumpy and irritable. We mutter about a rude driver and wonder why a normally friendly clerk is rushed and rude. A bothersome problem with a friend seems to be worse, and our boss is gruff and demanding. The people in our day reflect back to us our own rough mood.

Mirrors are useful in many different ways. There may be a person in our lives who irritates us or makes us angry, and they never seem to change. It could be something as small as a co-worker with a know-it-all attitude, or as difficult as a spouse who is domineering and controlling.

We know that asking others to change rarely works. Instead of just grumbling and complaining about them, we might ask: "Is what annoys me about this person mirroring back to me something I dislike in myself?"

I have asked this question many times and the answers have always given me insight, sometimes uncomfortably, into my own inner state.

An incident that happened years ago still reminds me of how effective mirrors are in revealing parts of oneself. I was in a meeting with a woman who was a specialist on grant proposal writing, and she was helping me write a proposal to fund a series of educational events on homelessness. It seemed that whenever I would ask her a question, she would not give me a clear answer. She would say, "Yes, this might be good information to include but it might make the proposal too long," or she would go into confusing explanations. I kept thinking, "You're the specialist, please just give me some clear direction."

I left our meeting totally frustrated, with no real understanding or plan for moving forward. As I later applied the mirror idea to myself, though, I almost laughed out loud. At the time, I had been going through a particularly indecisive and unclear time in my own life. No wonder I was irritated, and I was mostly irritated at myself. The mirror reflected back to me that I was the specialist in my own life, and I needed to get off the dime and make some much-needed decisions.

Interestingly, I was with the same woman a few years later in a similar situation, and she didn't irritate me at all. She hadn't changed, but I had. I was in a much better place.

Mirrors allow us to keep learning about ourselves. If we notice that we have people around us who consistently complain and are negative, what is that mirror saying about us? Is it time to shift from disliking their behavior to examining our own? Is the mirror telling us to become more positive, upbeat, and enjoyable to be around? Can we improve our lives by seeking out more positive people?

Doctors and health care professionals are especially powerful mirrors for our healing process. Am I irritated because my doctor, for instance, doesn't see me as a partner in my treatment? Do I get angry when he doesn't acknowledge the person I am behind my chronic illness? Is my irritation with my doctor a reflection of my irritation with myself for giving away my power over my own healing?

When I understand what the mirror is telling me, I might assert myself as a participant in my medical treatment and find that my doctor welcomes my involvement. Or perhaps I will seek another doctor who more closely matches my needs.

Sometimes it seems as if we live inside a mirrored egg, with reflections everywhere. And of course, as I learned in the seminar where my partner pointed out my strengths, our mirrors reflect our positives as well. When we are with people who care and who love us, it is a sure sign that we are loving toward ourselves and others. When we see the people around us enjoying and making the most of life, we are probably doing things that give ourselves satisfaction and contentment.

As we develop a better understanding of who and what we are, we can take more responsibility for our moods and attitudes. Rather than blaming others, we understand our own power to change our lives by changing things inside ourselves.

Each one of us is our own author. The stories we tell about our experiences are our creative expressions. As we grow to care more deeply about ourselves, our stories become less dependent on the ups and downs in our lives. As we become less critical, we find a growing stability because we are less swayed by what others think or do toward us. We rely more on our own internal guidance system, and our stories will reflect this.

Believing in ourselves is an evolving process. It requires shifts in the fundamentals of who we are, which doesn't happen overnight. It is something to which we commit and then watch as the ripples of change move slowly through ourselves and our surroundings. As our belief in ourselves takes hold, we see it when we feel affection for ourselves where in the past we would have taken ourselves to task, when the people around us gradually shift from judgmental to loving and encouraging, and when we comfortably cleave to decisions we know to be right even though those around us disagree.

We don't want to deny those parts of our personalities that need to be understood and worked on. At the same time, however, we want to hold close a realization that at our core we have a spiritual essence that is fueled by our love for ourselves. Then we can look at our stories and rewrite them with compassion and understanding.

Jamal Rahman, a Muslim and Sufi minister at the Interfaith Community Church in Seattle, wrote about his grandfather, a spiritual teacher who often spoke to his students about learning to be compassionate toward themselves. He would ask them to add a word of endearment to their names and to use that affectionate term whenever they talked to themselves. This practice, his grandfather said, allowed one's divine identity to step forward.

We are usually our own harshest critics. It's often much easier to make allowances for others' shortcomings than to forgive our own. Here are a few questions to help us see where we might want to extend more forgiveness and love toward ourselves:

❖ Do I often talk to myself negatively? Do I complain, criticize, and tell myself how inadequate I am? Would I like to speak to myself with a kinder, more loving voice?

❖ Do I feel as if I live two lives, one inside and one that I present to others? Would I like to be more honest and open?

❖ Do I often stretch the truth because I don't want to appear incompetent, or because I don't want to fail to live up to the expectations of others? Can I accept myself with less judgment and be more truthful about who I am?

❖ Am I comfortable receiving, whether it is a gift, a compliment, or affection? Do I want to become more comfortable with giving and receiving, so I can experience both with an open heart?

❖ Do I often feel alone, without spiritual connection? Do I want to grow in trust and in my relationship with my spirit?

CHAPTER 13

Strengthening Our Circle

"No man is the whole of himself. His friends are the rest of him."

RUTH SMALLEY, *GOOD LIFE ALMANAC*

When a crisis puts your feet to the fire, nothing can make the coals glow hotter than some of our relationships. I'm not sure I would have looked so deep inside if I hadn't been struggling with my arthritis at the same time that my marriage was collapsing.

Living with an illness can significantly change marriages and other important relationships. Some relationships fall apart, while others become deeper. The challenges of tough experiences embolden some couples to live their lives together with more meaning, reshaping and clarifying what is important. But in my marriage, stress from my illness highlighted weaknesses that had accumulated under the surface for many years.

Often it's not so much the nature of a stressful situation as how we react that determines the outcome. My response to the stress of being sick was to hide and repress my fears and uncertainties.

Before my illness, I believed that a strong person was self-sufficient, neither asking for nor needing anything from others. With the onset of arthritis, that belief no longer worked for me. There was too much pain; too much confusion; too many areas where I needed to ask for help from my family. But I didn't know how to reach out and express myself, how to ask for help or to listen to what my husband and sons were feeling.

I knew it wasn't just me who had difficulty coping—we were all feeling lost in those early years of my illness. It was clear to my family that every day I was becoming more physically limited in what I could do. We were all hurt when I could no longer share in many of the activities we used to do together. But throughout those wrenching changes, we acted as if nothing had happened. The changes in our lives that flowed from my arthritis were buried in silence.

It never occurred to me, for instance, to ask my husband what he was feeling. Discussing emotions or personal needs did not come naturally to either of us, so it had not been a normal part of our marriage. As a consequence, the difficult but necessary conversations didn't happen. While we both suppressed our thoughts and emotions, my body became more locked down with arthritis.

Unfortunately this behavior seemed familiar and normal. It was similar to the feelings of isolation I had had as a young teen-ager, living in a family unable to express the anguish around my mother's illness and death. I was back in that same place.

As I drifted into the troubled waters of illness and divorce, I gradually began to understand that my resentment and frustration were messengers that told me important things. It dawned on me that rather than being suppressed, those negative feelings should be acknowledged and dealt with. They are part of being alive, good indicators of what we need but lack. I also noticed that as I accepted my feelings, I became more comfortable listening to and talking about other people's emotions.

Although the anger and frustration were useful indicators, I knew I didn't want them to become dominant emotions. When they rose to the surface, I began to consciously acknowledge them and then choose to replace them with uplifting thoughts that would lead toward more positive feelings.

At the same time I started welcoming my feelings, I noticed that there were mental barriers against expressing them. A recurring thought was that expressing my innermost dark emotions would make matters worse. They would judge me. I remembered times when I had expressed my feelings and regretted it because of the consequences. Also, deep inside, I wanted to stay in a false comfort zone.

I posed questions to myself to help me speak up about my feelings. What would happen if I expressed them, without worrying about the consequences? Then I reminded myself of people over the years with whom I could have deep, caring conversations on any subject. These positive scenarios helped me communicate more of my feelings, even if I didn't know exactly what I would say or how it would be received.

I learned skills to express myself more clearly and honestly. "I" statements, for instance, help a person talk about their feelings without blaming others. I worked on simply describing situations by how they make me feel, rather than slipping into telling others what they should do.

Instead of saying "You should help me," for example, I might say "I need help at dinner time. Preparing and cleaning up are really difficult for me." This may sound like a formula without spontaneity, but after some practice it comes naturally. It makes it easier to own and express one's feelings and needs, and allows the other person to hear you without defensiveness.

At the bottom of all this was an important truth. I can't control the outcome of conversations, but I can stay true to myself. When my communication is honest and heartfelt, what follows will be for the best.

The pain of my divorce gave me the incentive to break out of my old ways and create new patterns of openness about my feelings. The results changed my heart and paved the way for a loving partner to walk into my life some years later.

Someone once said to me that in order to get clear about the kind of future partner you want, it helps to list his qualities you would like. When I thought about what I wanted in a relationship, the first thought that came to mind was fun loving. My life was way too serious. After that I wrote down other qualities that were important to me: a commitment to our love, an openness in sharing feelings, and an adventurous nature. I thought about the people around me, and nobody quite seemed to fit.

At some point, it became clear that before I could attract someone who had the attributes I wanted in a partner, I first had to have those qualities myself. With that in mind, I watched how I behaved. When I started holding back emotionally, I reminded myself that if I wanted to have a man in my life who openly discussed his feelings, I had to be more open.

I made a concerted effort to look on the amusing side of things, even of serious situations. As I worked at enhancing my humor, I found that I liked myself more. I enjoyed my own company. Energy of change was in the air. I was opening up to new experiences.

A few years later I was at a photography exhibition and bumped into Tim, an old friend. We were both surprised that after all the years since we had worked together on an environmental project, we still had much in common. We eventually married, and it's not surprising that he has the qualities that I had written down.

Interestingly, Tim told me that he had had a similar experience. Because a friend at work asked him what kind of person he was looking for in a relationship, he wrote down a list of attributes. When he showed his list to his friend, she said, "I think you should add the quality of emotional strength. It would be good for you to find someone you can lean on, rather than continuing your pattern of being around people who lean on you." Despite the fact that we hadn't seen each other in years, he said that I had spontaneously come to mind.

The same process works just as well with other people in our lives. Listing the attributes we like is a good way to attract people who possess them. If we want friends who are understanding and fun or doctors who are caring and open to new ideas, it is good to list those characteristics and keep them in mind. It also helps, sometimes, to share our lists with a friend, because old patterns can block us from seeing potential aspects of people from whom we would benefit. Finally, of course, we need to bring those things forth in ourselves.

Most of us tend to look outward for change whenever we feel something lacking in our lives, rather than putting our energies toward improving ourselves. This is true whether we are seeking a loving partner, meaningful friendships, or even a different job. Significant positive change almost always starts on the inside, with outward results following. It also helps, of course, to have some specifics in mind about the changes we want. The clearer we are about what we want, the better will be the results we attract.

Illness can throw our relationships off kilter. Roles and routines change, and change can be wrenching. We may get so absorbed in our emotional and physical pain that we yearn for others to rescue us. Fearful and frustrated, we lose sight of how our personalities may be changing.

We may think that the world isn't fair. We become more demanding. Or we withdraw from others, ignoring how important it is to give appreciation for help and support. We may slip into a pattern of constant complaints.

Resentment and criticism may dominate our conversations. It's too hot or cold; the doctors are not good; people don't seem to care or come around any more. Before we know it, our world mirrors our complaints.

This is a situation where our observer voice can be helpful. If we listen to our observer, we'll become aware that we have slipped into a sour disposition. If we follow that awareness with the intent to change, we can gradually reverse the negativity and open our hearts more fully to others. As with any major change it doesn't happen easily or quickly, but as we take the first steps and our lives brighten, we find ourselves naturally wanting to continue moving forward.

It's also a good thing to remember that even if we stay as positive, appreciative, and upbeat as we can, almost everyone who faces chronic illness grapples with adjusting their support system to their new situation.

I asked my friend Fran how she strengthened her circle of support after she was diagnosed with breast cancer. Here are some of her thoughts:

I remember choosing to be with friends who had "good energy," people who were supportive with humor and practical help, and open to difficult conversations. I avoided friends who challenged the treatment choices I was making, who felt the need to tell me about worst cases, who had ideas about what caused my cancer, or who were obviously very fearful about cancer for themselves.

In addition, there were some people who simply withdrew from our friendship. Maybe they couldn't handle their own fears or anxieties about cancer or related issues. Maybe my illness was a reminder of those fears. If so, there was nothing that I could do to comfort them or allay their discomfort.

I did reach out to several long-time women friends who lived far away, but who had known me since my children were very young. We had long telephone conversations and exchanged letters. We could talk comfortably about my family, treatment, and surgery, and I never felt I had to protect them from what I was feeling. I could practice saying things to them that I wanted to say to family members or doctors. They were always there, not to judge but to listen and reflect back what they were hearing and to challenge me in supportive ways.

My husband Reed was different. He did not do the same kind of reaching out to friends. He talked about feeling like an outsider to what I was going through, and of not feeling in any systematic way that he was being helpful. He said that most of what he did was improvised, and he wasn't confident that what he was doing was the right thing.

Reed also realized that he had his own fear, and he knew that we had to talk about our fears and be open and honest about our feelings. We had to admit to each other and to ourselves how scared we were.

Six years after my first bout of cancer I was diagnosed with breast cancer again, and the treatment included a mastectomy. The second occurrence really knocked the ground out from under us, but this time we quickly acknowledged our deepest fears to one another.

The two experiences with cancer have been touchstones for how we want to live our lives, demonstrating our love and commitment to one another and making decisions about our future based on our desire to live as fully as we can.

For both Reed and me there is a particular joy in connecting with each other and with other people in ways we would never have dreamed possible before suffering those hard times. After all that, we are far more able and willing to share our feelings about our experiences and about what we have learned.

Fears of an unknown future caused Fran and Reed to reshape their lives. When Fran was in the throes of cancer, they both participated in a wellness program they found very helpful, and for many years after her illness they continued in the program as volunteers. They now offer some of what they learned to others, leading free classes on breath and tai chi in our small community.

The true essence of support doesn't go just one way; it flows back and forth. When both giving and receiving come from our hearts, they are two sides of the same coin. Whether we are open-heartedly giving or receiving with gratitude, we are blessed by the presence of the gift.

Support systems come in many forms, but most important are the assurance and support we give to ourselves. One way that I consistently support myself is by creating a circle of love. I sit quietly and visualize people I love sitting with me in a circle. It surprises me sometimes who seems to want to be there; my father, who passed away several years ago, is always present. As we sit quietly together, I visualize a band of white light connecting our hearts. The heart circle flows through us as a stream of calm and peace, and it fills me with abiding support. When I am there, I am awash in the feeling that all those loving souls are wishing the very best for me.

Some days it's a challenge to stay open to giving and to receiving. But I do know this—when I allow my heart to reach out to another, a small miracle happens. In those precious moments, love lifts me up.

There is an old story about the nature of heaven and hell. It seems a disciple of a wise teacher had grown very concerned about what these two places were really like and how they differed, so the teacher took the disciple and descended into the depths of hell.

They came to a great room with thousands of people all seated at a vast banquet table. The table was overflowing with an endless variety of delicious foods. Each person was provided with a fork, but there was a problem—all the forks were three feet long. This, of course, made it impossible to get the food from the table to their mouths, and consequently even in the presence of bountiful food, everyone was starving.

Then the teacher took the disciple to heaven. They came to a great room with thousands of people all seated at a banquet table identical to the one they had seen in hell. Again the table was overflowing with the finest foods, and also as in hell, each person had a fork that was three feet long. The difference, however, was that here, rather than starving because they couldn't get the food from the table into their own mouths, they were using their long forks to feed each other.

Literally and figuratively, reaching out to others strengthens them and us.

CHAPTER 14

Beginner's Mind

"And thus the world is full of leaves and feathers, and comfort, and instruction."

MARY OLIVER, FROM THE POEM, "CROW"

We have no idea what our future holds but when we maintain a sincere wish to grow, growth will happen because we carry the seeds of it inside us. As we learn this, we develop trust in our path and relax. We push less and meander more. We gradually open to a deeper sense of wholeness among all the facets of our being.

Our mental, emotional, physical, and spiritual parts are dynamically intertwined. Stress in one area stresses the others, and health in one promotes health in the others. We can feel a distinct difference between times when these aspects are in harmony with each other and when they are not.

There will be times in our chronic illness when we lose our balance on a tide of emotions, or believe that our rational mind is the only guide we can rely on to get us through. If we know the feeling and value of being in harmony, however, we can bring ourselves back to center.

Our minds are particularly skillful at dominating our other aspects, and our schooling has taught us that we should only rely on things that are rational and externally verifiable. Eckhart Tolle, in his book, *Stillness Speaks*, describes the challenge of the dominant mind: "The stream of thinking has enormous momentum that can easily drag you along with it. Every thought pretends that it matters so much. It wants to draw your attention in completely."

If we understand our patterns, we can bring ourselves back into balance. When we are aware that difficult times trigger an array of automatic responses, we take a big step toward breaking out of the recurring loop of pain, struggle, and more pain. When we practice inserting our positive beliefs into the stream of negative thoughts, the stream shifts and the current weakens. We can move from feeling that every mental and emotional reaction is true, to knowing the truth of our centers. We can gentle our emotional storms and bend our thoughts into more positive and hopeful channels.

Our thoughts can then become more our friends than our enemies, and we can better align our minds, emotions, spirits, and bodies to assist whatever part of us is in need. Our body fear subsides. Our illness fades into something about us, not the definition of who we are. We take an enormous step along our healing path when we understand how much power we have within ourselves to feel better.

There is great reward when all our aspects are working in harmony. We can maintain caring relationships with our bodies, even when we're in pain and discomfort. Rather than distancing ourselves we will stay with our bodies, as we would with a friend in times of trouble.

When we more fully understand that growing and expanding our consciousness is something we can do, we acquire power over our lives. We are less inclined to blame others or hard luck or anything else for our situations and experiences. We realize that in the most significant ways, we are our own creators. We will experience momentous losses and cruel circumstances, but we know that how we respond to them and weave them into the context of our lives are within our control.

As we guide our internal lives more positively through difficult times, we discover that external aspects of our lives improve as well.

We are attracted to people who care about growing into their own wholeness. We gravitate to relationships where there is a beneficial exchange of pleasure, understanding, and unconditional love.

We don't have to play roles to win acceptance. We are more honest and true to ourselves. Our significant relationships deepen because we are able to go beyond the trivialities of day-to-day events. Resentments fade when hearts are open to connection with our spirit.

We also become aware of relationships that lessen us, stifle and suffocate us. We realize we have choices about whom we want around us. We look honestly inside to see if we are lessening others. Most importantly, we ask whether our troubling relationships are mirroring something we would like to change within ourselves.

We become less judgmental and more forgiving. We no longer have to be imprisoned in the tiresome stories we played and replayed from the past. We understand that we will never know all aspects of the events and people that brought us resentment and hurt, but we are willing to release their dark shadows.

As we become more quiet and contemplative, we begin to hear a whisper inside calling us to nurture our inner beings. We may respond in a variety of ways: from creating times of prayer or meditation, to finding a community of people who share similar aspirations, or to seeking more contact with the natural world.

Many of us naturally gravitate toward nature as we grow. It fosters our stillness and expands our sense of connection to everything that exists outside us. When we are transfixed by a chattering squirrel, the beauty of a bright flower, or wind through the branches of a majestic tree, we experience healing unity.

Even when we cannot go outside, our imaginations can travel there. That can be enough to elevate our spirits and help our egos diminish into the background.

In Buddhism there is a concept of the beginner's mind. It is the opposite of unconsciously living in rote and routine. A beginner's mind allows us to approach life with a desire to be astonished by wonder and beauty. We hold ourselves vulnerable to surprising possibilities and new perspectives.

A Buddhist friend, Roger, shared his story of learning about the beginner's mind this way:

In his book, Zen Mind, Beginner's Mind, *the Zen master Shunryu Suzuki describes this desirable approach to life as being centered in the moment. I understand his concept of beginner's mind as a sort of a childlike openness.*

Perhaps Jesus had something similar in mind when he said, "I tell you the truth, unless you change and become like little children, you will never enter the kingdom of heaven." There are probably a lot of different ways to understand this beginner's mind. Perhaps a herd of buffalo will help.

I first met my own Zen master, Reverend Saito, Head Minister of the Buddhist Temple of Chicago, forty years ago when he came to our Midwestern university to lecture during World Religion Week.

At the end of the week as I was driving him to the airport, we chanced to approach a state park. Grazing in the field was a herd of about twelve buffalo. I pulled over and stopped so we could get out and look at them.

Reverend Saito suddenly appeared childlike with wonder. His eyes got big, having never seen a buffalo before. He was astonished; it was obviously a magical moment for him. We never discussed the experience.

Twenty-five years later, I was at my teacher's bed in a hospital in Hawaii—he was dying. He had been unable to make conversation for several hours. Suddenly he opened his eyes and his face brightened. Looking at the hospital ceiling as if it were a bridge across time, he uttered the last word I ever heard from him—"buffalo." It was his final teaching.

Whenever I think of that moment I feel deeply what Suzuki meant when he wrote about the beginner's mind.

The labyrinth of this book has wound around, here and there, through my own life lessons and experiences of others on their healing paths. I hope you have experienced it that way: a series of trusting steps that, even though they do not follow a consistent spiral, move toward a center.

We are at the end, but like all endings this is also a beginning. May we all have beginners' minds as we embrace our continuing lives and the profound healing possibilities they contain. When we grow, all aspects of us deepen and expand. We become more alive and aware, layer-by-layer.

Here is a gentle meditation:

Float with me on the surface of a bright clear stream meandering through a high mountain meadow.

We are on a small raft and the current flows under us, gently guiding us on our path of water.

There are solid and unmoving boulders in the stream, and the water bubbles and gurgles as it swirls around them.

Our raft drifts easily and safely by the boulders, and we take a slow deep breath and sink into relaxation.

We trust the water that flows under and around us, buoying us up. Our thoughts are still. We allow ourselves to become one with the current.

We fill with trust and contentment as we drift along beneath the clear blue sky.

We are traveling together this river of life.

APPENDIX 1

Embracing Change Practices

*H*ere are the exercises you encountered in the book. They work best if you can find your way to a quiet comfortable place where you won't be interrupted. No matter what your setting though, if you are in a crisis, a period of anxiety or depression, or want to gain more energy, they can help.

Finger Labyrinth (Introduction)

Whether you walk a labyrinth or move through one with your finger, they are wonderful tools for encouraging the mind to release control and the heart to trust.

Turn to the labyrinth picture at the end of the Introduction. Clear your mind, slow and deepen your breath, and allow your body to relax. Slide your finger into the labyrinth entrance and allow it to slowly follow the path, as if you were meandering through a large labyrinth in a grassy field. As your finger wends its way in and out and in again, allow yourself to begin releasing something you no longer wish to carry in your life. Pause at the center of the labyrinth and breathe into the light empty space you are creating. Move slowly back toward the entrance, bringing lightness and clarity with you.

Getting to Know Your Body Fear (Chapter Two)

Take some time to consider what fears you have about your body. Write them down if you wish. On balance, do you see your body as something to fear? Does the uncertainty of what's going to happen to you in the future leave you feeling helpless and scared?

Now consider the words you use to describe certain areas of your body, especially those particularly affected by your illness. Do you find yourself talking about "my bad back" or "my weak stomach?" Do these words contain clues to your true feelings about your body?

Changing Body Fear into Trust (Chapter Two)

Sit quietly and ease into a deep and comfortable breathing rhythm. Let your mind fill with familiar fears about your body. Conjure up all the scary things that might happen. Imagine the worst, and allow your thoughts to keep coming.

Ride the waves of emotion as they build until slowly, after two or three minutes, the intensity begins to dissipate. Move back into an easy breathing rhythm.

Go into your memory to a time when your body felt strong and healthy. Let yourself dwell on feeling truly good in your body, and hold the sensation in this moment. Feel your hands tingle and wiggle your toes. Sink into your breathing and feel the rhythm of your chest rising and falling. Take time to relish this feeling.

Affirm your intent to replace fears about your body with your knowledge of its innate strength and resilience, its healing intelligence. Although you don't have all the answers, know that you will work with your body to help it move toward health. Again, take time to be with those good feelings.

Finally, picture yourself with light flooding your whole body.

Visualize your feet firm on the earth, as if you are a great oak tree with deep abiding roots. Relax into the safety the moment holds.

Using Conscious Breathing (Chapter Three)

Begin by placing your tongue just behind your teeth on the roof of your mouth. Quietly inhale through your nose, and exhale noisily through your mouth. The sound you want to make when you exhale is a kind of whoosh.

Inhale again through your nose to a count of four, hold your breath to a count of seven, and exhale through your mouth to a count of eight. As you exhale through your mouth, try to rid yourself completely of all the air in your lungs.

Repeat your breathing cycle four times. If you can, do this several times a day. At first you may feel light-headed, but you will soon adjust to the increased oxygen.

Once you have practiced this four-seven-eight rhythm for a while, you will no longer need to keep track by counting. It will come naturally as you follow your breath with your mind, and experience the expanded energy and peace that follow.

You can use your breath exercise whenever you want to calm yourself down, raise your energy, or diminish pain.

Releasing Agitation (Chapter Four)

Close your eyes and connect with your body by taking deep slow breaths. Visualize a band of white light circling clockwise around you. Allow yourself to feel the spinning circle of light.

Next, imagine reversing the band of light so it rotates around you in the opposite direction, counter-clockwise. Once the light is turning easily, gently push your agitation and worry into the light, which flings it out and away.

Stay with this, gently breathing, until your agitation and the emotion that caused it are gone. Bring your band of light back into a comforting clockwise circle around you, and sink into its ease.

Using Intuition (Chapter Five)

The next time you are trying to make a hard decision, hold the issue close to you. Imagine it as a homing pigeon you are about to release. Ask yourself for direction toward your highest good. Picture releasing the pigeon and sending it deep within your spirit. See it spreading its wings to gather wisdom.

Over the next few days, watch for an answer. It may come in a dream, as a sudden insight, an off-hand remark by a friend, something you read or see, or in some other way. It may happen immediately or it may take longer, but when the time is right, your answer will find its way back to you.

Blowing Negativity Away (Chapter Six)

The next time someone says something rude or does something hurtful to you, imagine their action as a wind blowing through you, leaving you untouched.

Breathe slowly and deeply into any knots and tensions, and feel them gradually ease and release.

When you return to the moment, notice how quieted and peaceful you are. Take a deep breath and center yourself in your balance.

Preparing for Sleep (Chapter Eight)

Get comfortable in bed, turn off the light, and close your eyes. Picture yourself standing under a gentle waterfall, a beautiful natural place with pastel flowers and green foliage surrounding cascading water.

Slowly take deep breaths as you absorb the sights and sounds around you. Listen to the sound of the gently tumbling water. As the water flows over you, feel it cleanse and soothe your body from head to toe.

While you are standing beneath the flowing stream of water, slowly scan your body. When you find a tight place, gently breathe into the tenseness to release it and allow the water to carry it away.

Visualize the water washing away all your cares, until you feel free and transparent. Your breath relaxes even more. You are ready to slip gently into sleep.

Finding Healing Connections (Chapter Nine)

We each have great power to increase our health, reduce our discomfort, and improve our attitude by establishing and enhancing our healing connections. Here are a few questions to ask yourself as you think about the healing connections in your life:

❖ Do I often enjoy a good laugh or make someone else laugh or smile?
❖ Do I often reach out to touch others in need?
❖ Do I take heart from those around me who show courage?
❖ Am I around people who are generally positive and upbeat and see the best in me? Do I see the best in them?

If you answered "no" to some of these questions, you might want to create opportunities that will allow you to change your answers. Identify some healing connections—people, activities, animals, plants, places—that will strengthen and enrich your life, and then make those connections.

Opening to Possibilities (Chapter Ten)

Go to a quiet, comfortable place. Close your eyes and relax into your breathing. Feel your body and mind at ease and receptive.

Think about a troubling situation in your life. Allow thoughts and feelings to come to the surface. Are they all worried, anxious, negative? Are there some among them that are hopeful, open to new opportunities?

If there are positive thoughts, bring them to the front of your mind. Imagine other hopeful aspects of the situation and bring those into your mind as well.

Remind yourself that a troubling situation often can have a positive outcome because of possibilities that you never thought of or anticipated.

Focus on your breath and hold the troubling situation gently in your mind, surrounded by hope and awareness of possible positive outcomes.

Release the situation from your mind, breathe easily, and open your eyes.

Each day, practice believing impossible things.

Showing Appreciation (Chapter Eleven)

Find a quiet place where you are alone.

Close your eyes and follow your breath as it flows easily in and out.

Place your hand over your heart and feel its steady beat.

Expand your heart to include a circle of caring people in your life.

Imagine one special person from the circle coming forward, and feel your hearts connect.

Appreciate all that person is to you.

Breathe in the grateful feelings and the loving connection.

Rest awhile in the glow of gratitude.

The next time you are with that person, give voice to your feelings.

Deepening Self-Love and Forgiveness (Chapter Twelve)

We are usually our own harshest critics. It's often much easier to make allowances for others' shortcomings than to forgive our own. Here are a few questions to help us see where we might want to extend more forgiveness and love toward ourselves:

- ❖ Do I often talk to myself negatively? Do I complain, criticize, and tell myself how inadequate I am? Would I like to speak to myself with a kinder, more loving voice?
- ❖ Do I feel as if I live two lives, one inside and one that I present to others? Would I like to be more honest and open?
- ❖ Do I often stretch the truth because I don't want to appear incompetent, or because I don't want to fail to live up to the expectations of others? Can I accept myself with less judgment and be more truthful about who I am?
- ❖ Am I comfortable receiving, whether it is a gift, a compliment, or affection? Do I want to become more comfortable with giving and receiving, so I can experience both with an open heart?
- ❖ Do I often feel alone, without spiritual connection? Do I want to grow in trust and in my relationship with my spirit?

Visualizing a Circle of Love (Chapter Thirteen)

Sit quietly and visualize people you love sitting with you in a circle. In addition to the ones that come quickly to mind, it will sometimes surprise you who wants to be there. Perhaps a parent or friend who passed away, a companion who walked with you during a difficult time, or someone you haven't thought of in a long time, may appear.

As you sit quietly together, visualize a band of white light connecting your hearts. The heart circle flows through all of you as a stream of calm and peace, and it fills you with abiding support. Allow yourself to be awash in the feeling that all those loving souls are wishing the very best for you.

Gently Down the Stream (Chapter Fourteen)

Here is a gentle meditation to feel peace:

See yourself floating on the surface of a bright clear stream meandering through a high mountain meadow.
You are on a small raft and the current flows under you, gently guiding you on your path of water.
There are solid and unmoving boulders in the stream, and the water bubbles and gurgles as it swirls around them.
Your raft drifts easily and safely by the boulders, and you take a slow deep breath and sink into relaxation.
You trust the water that flows under and around you, buoying you up.
Your thoughts are still. You allow yourself to become one with the current.
You fill with trust and contentment as you drift along beneath the clear blue sky.
You are traveling the river of life.

APPENDIX 2
Annotated Bibliography

On Death and Dying by Elizabeth Kubler-Ross (Tavistock Publications Limited, 1970).

The grieving stages that Kubler-Ross outlined in this landmark book are as respected and applicable today as they were when they were written over four decades ago.

In the chaotic beginnings of my illness, her book provided me with a much-needed framework for understanding more clearly the emotional roller coaster I was riding. Her grief stages still resonate for me throughout times of loss. (Chapter One)

Magical Mind, Magical Body by Deepak Chopra M.D. (CD series, Nightingale Conant, 1991).

Chopra skillfully illuminates the large concept of how the mind/body connection functions with specifics, such as how all 50 trillion cells in our bodies actively participate in our thoughts. The mind/body connection gives us enormous personal power to channel our thoughts in a healing direction.

While listening to Chopra, I was struck with how important it is to remember and affirm that there is a constant river of intelligence that flows within us, that is always available. This lasting connection with our inner intelligence is where our true potential for healing resides. (Chapter Two)

Breathing: The Master Key to Self-Healing by Andrew Weil M.D. (audio CD collection, Sounds True, 2000).

Dr. Weil so believes in the importance of breath to health and healing that if he had to give just one bit of healing advice, it would be to learn how to breathe correctly. This CD contains a series of simple breathing exercises, and connects them to the benefits they provide.

The use of breath for connection among my body, mind, and spirit continues to be fundamental to my self-healing. I use my breath to talk to my body, and as a gentle reminder to stay in the present and put brakes on negative thoughts. (Chapter Three)

You Can Heal Your Life by Louise Hay (Hay House, 2004).

Louise Hay connects belief systems to specific physical illnesses. Through affirmations and other tools, Louise Hay guides people to bring unconscious and unhealthy mental patterns to the surface, so they can be examined and changed.

This book helped me realize that my life had been heavily based on the needs of others rather than myself, and that changing this pattern could be a significant healing force with my rheumatoid arthritis. (Chapter Four)

I Will Not Die an Unlived Life: Reclaiming Purpose and Passion by Dawna Markova (Conari Press, 2000).

Dawna Markova was diagnosed with cancer and as a result decided to take a six-month retreat to the mountains of Utah for rest and reflection. This poetic narrative chronicles her inner search for passion and meaning in her life. (Chapter Four)

The Path of Transformation: How Healing Ourselves Can Change the World by Shaki Gawain (Nataraj Publishing, revised edition, 2000).

Shaki Gawain is a pioneer whose books on healing focus on the importance of a spiritual path to personal growth. She believes that being committed to our own spiritual growth gives our lives meaning, and emphasizes the deep contribution each of our life journeys has to the earth's healing. (Chapter Four)

Molecules of Emotion: The Science Behind Mind-Body Medicine
by Candace Pert Ph.D. (Scribner, 2003).

Although most of us conceive of our minds as a function of our brains, Pert's pioneering research demonstrates how our thoughts and feelings are to a great extent created by a complex interaction of chemical messengers throughout our bodies. She calls this unification of our mind, emotions, and spirit with our physical body, the "bodymind."

Woven throughout is her personal story as a female scientist struggling to develop and disseminate new concepts in a competitive and rigidly hierarchical system. (Chapter Five)

Forgive for Good: A Proven Prescription for Health and Happiness
by Fred Luskin Ph.D. (HarperCollins 2003).

We know that learning how to forgive is good medicine for our bodies, because they carry the burden of grievances as strongly as do our hearts and minds. Luskin believes that when a person understands how a grievance is formed, they are better able to heal. He teaches how to forgive, and how to create a meaningful story of our life experiences. (Chapter Six)

A Joseph Campbell Companion: Reflections on the Art of Living
by Diane K. Osborn (Harper Perennial, 1991).

The author combines excerpts from Campbell's works into an inspiring book on myths that give us courage to follow "a hero's journey." Campbell is a master at identifying common threads of wisdom throughout civilizations, and expressing them powerfully and succinctly. A good example is, "We must be willing to let go of the life we planned so as to have the life that is waiting for us."

Another excellent way to begin the journey with Joseph Campbell is to listen to the audio version of *Joseph Campbell and the Power of Myth*, a conversation between Joseph Campbell and Bill Moyers (audio CD, HighBridge Audio, 2001). (Chapter Seven)

Time Shifting: Creating More Time to Enjoy Your Life by Stephan Rechtschaffen, M.D. (Doubleday, 1996).

We automatically think of time as fixed and objective, but Rechtschaffen teaches that time is subjective, and that we can take control of our lives by the way we think about time. In this fascinating book he encourages his readers to create a new relationship with time, one that positively affects their sense of well-being through conscious expansion of the moment. *Time Shifting* contains simple and practical ways to change the way time works in our lives. (Chapter Eight)

Let Your Life Speak: Listening for the Voice of Vocation by Parker J. Palmer (Jossey-Bass, 2000).

I found Palmer's self- exploration and the depression and closed doors he experienced particularly poignant and similar to early struggles I faced with chronic illness. His book reminds us that whatever our life struggle might be, at the core is the need to learn to love ourselves. (Chapter Twelve)

The Voice of Knowledge: A Practical Guide to Inner Peace by Don Miguel Ruiz (Amber-Allen, 2004).

Ruiz focuses on the fact that that the "knowledge" given to us by parents and teachers of how to live in the world and to be "good" and "successful," is often not only wrong, but poisonous. The poison acts by splitting us off from what we naturally knew as children—how to live in the moment and express who we truly are. This inspiring book guides and supports its readers to recover and celebrate their authentic selves. (Chapter Twelve)

Stillness Speaks by Eckhart Tolle (New World Library and Namaste, 2003).

Tolle has become a worldwide phenomenon because of his simple profundity. This quiet little book is chock-full of his wise teachings, arranged in short segments that allow the reader to move slowly and take in its gifts. As Tolle says in his introduction, "Allow the book to do its work, to awaken you from the old grooves of your repetitive and conditional thinking." It does that and much more. (Chapter Fourteen)

CPSIA information can be obtained at www.ICGtesting.com
Printed in the USA
LVOW100354201012

303666LV00003B/3/P